nic
4.50

D1279972

FATIGUE

Mechanism and Management

Publication Number 621

AMERICAN LECTURE SERIES®

A Monograph in

AMERICAN LECTURES IN LIVING CHEMISTRY

Edited by

I. NEWTON KUGELMASS, M.D. Ph.D., Sc.D.

Consultant to the Departments of Health and Hospitals
New York, New York

FATIGUE

Mechanism and Management

By

S. HOWARD BARTLEY

Professor of Psychology
Michigan State University
East Lansing, Michigan

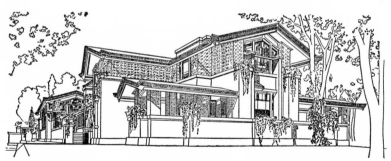

CHARLES C THOMAS • PUBLISHER

Springfield • Illinois • U.S.A.

Published and Distributed Throughout the World by

CHARLES C THOMAS • PUBLISHER

BANNERSTONE HOUSE

301-327 East Lawrence Avenue, Springfield, Illinois, U.S.A.

NATCHEZ PLANTATION HOUSE

735 North Atlantic Boulevard, Fort Lauderdale, Florida, U.S.A.

With THOMAS BOOKS careful attention is given to all details of manufacturing and design. It is the Publisher's desire to present books that are satisfactory as to their physical qualities and artistic possibilities and appropriate for their particular use. THOMAS BOOKS will be true to those laws of quality that assure a good name and good will.

Printed in the United States of America

W-2

To

David Bruce Dill

A monumental worker in the study

of human performance

Foreword

Our Living Chemistry Series was conceived by
Editor and Publisher to advance the newer
knowledge of chemical medicine in the cause of clinical practice.
The interdependence of chemistry and medicine is so great that
physicians are turning to chemistry, and chemists to medicine in
order to understand the underlying basis of life processes in
health and disease. Once chemical truths, proofs and convictions
become sound foundations for clinical phenomena, key hybrid
investigators clarify the bewildering panorama of biochemical
progress for application in everyday practice, stimulation of
experimental research, and extension of postgraduate instruction.
Each of our monographs thus unravels the chemical mechanisms
and clinical management of many diseases that have remained
relatively static in the minds of medical men for three thousand
years. Our new Series is charged with the *nisus élan* of chemical
wisdom, supreme in choice of international authors, optimal in
standards of chemical scholarship, provocative in imagination
for experimental research, comprehensive in discussions of
scientific medicine, and authoritative in chemical perspective
of human disorders.

Dr. Bartley of Michigan unravels fatigue in perspicuous
thoughts on the psychic and physiological phenomena that
violate the biological unity of the integrated self. The state of
the body at any moment is the resultant of vectorial forces main-
taining a dynamic equilibrium for optimal functioning. When
the body is subjected to stress there is a new alignment of altered
forces and a new position of equilibrium established. But
manifestations of fatigue herald the failure of the body to main-

tain an equilibrial condition or an exaggeration of the forces involved in the equilibrium. The threatened disorganization of the disturbed individual evokes tension which exceeds the normal coping devices of the organism, hence special mechanisms are called upon to maintain the equilibrium at a lower level of total functioning with the best possible façade at minimal discomfort. This suboptimal state can be reversed by specific therapy evaluated for each type of fatigue according to the underlying mechanism.

Beard (1869) established the concept of neurasthenia; Da Costa (1871), neurocirculatory asthenia; Weir Mitchell (1872), functional neurosis. Mosso (1884) developed the ergograph to measure the decrement in muscle ability to contract fully when repeatedly stimulated. Freud (1890) described psychic fatigue. Rivers (1896) demonstrated that practice and fatigue and rest and fatigue are mutually antagonistic and a warming-up period after work improves performance. McDougal (1905) observed the diurnal performance rhythm. Wells (1912) found decreased performance masked by increased effort to achieve the same results. Smith (1916) could not correlate subjective feelings with objective output. Bills (1931) revealed that transient mental block of inactivity increased in frequency with continuous performance until the work accomplished was nil. Browne (1949) showed that performance increases as environment reaches the optimal biological range. Dill (1950) delineated the patterns of fatigue with respective prevention procedures. Bartley (1957) formulated the clinical concept of psychologic fatigue.

Fatigue is the most frequent yet the most obstruse of all symptoms in everyday practice with many equivalents—tiredness, weakness, exhaustion, lassitude or lack of energy—each possessing some essential distinction but all denoting the same sort of sensation. It may be viewed as physiological changes in internal organs reflected as an overt behavior disorder in work decrement or as psychological changes manifested in personal dissatisfaction. Fatigue is a "whole" symptom felt throughout the body, not confined to special regions or specific functions, emanating from the whole of body and mind, an interrelationship that governs the consciousness of tiredness. Natural fatigue is a protective phenomenon that helps maintain the equilibrium of the organism by stimulating the desire for natural restoratives—food and rest— a condition to be desired rather than feared for life without stress is unhealthy. The purpose of fatigue is self-preservation of self-esteem not merely protection against physical injury. It is not a negative goal, a lack of energy but an unconscious desire for inactivity. There is a reciprocal relationship between fatigue and anxiety, both protective devices but the one is inactivity and the other a call for positive action to extricate one's self from a predicament.

Psychoneurotic fatigue is worse in the morning but improves as the day progresses. A patient feels like lying down but cannot sleep. The feeling of fatigue related to certain activities and special events for initiation of activity is difficult and capacity for work reduced. Persistent fatigue leads to failure of the recuperating powers, the resulting exhaustion activating a latent disease process or precipitating a pathological disorder. Extreme exhaustion makes a patient incapable of the least exacting work as a result of constitutional inadequacy with shallow reserves readily depleted. So much energy is wasted in careless activity, fits of temper and riots of emotion that insufficient energy remains for the serious business of life. Rest is the worst treatment, for with work, fatigue disappears. It is stagnation that must be removed. Chronic fatigue per se reveals neither physical signs nor abnormalities, except in myasthenia, diabetes, tuberculosis, Addison's disease, myxedema, severe anemia, glomerulonephritis, chronic infection, cardiac insufficiency, or malignancy, each of which has distinctive clinical features. Those affected are naturally importunate in the expectation of some removable cause or alternately the provision of an energizer or substitute for inherent deficiency.

Blood of a fatigued individual injected into a rested one produces the overt manifestations of fatigue. It is characterized by tremulous muscle action, clumsy movements, accelerated breathing, quickening pulse, increased pulse pressure, elevated

blood pressure, increased metabolism, decreased blood glucose
and leucocytosis. Physiological changes include depletion of
muscle glycogen, accumulation of lactic acid and other metabo-
lites interfering with prolonged contractility and muscle recovery. Exhaustion of metabolic reserves is paralleled by
limitation of the cardiovascular and respiratory systems reflecting
innate individual differences in the energy potential of human
beings. The human machine represented by the trinity DNA,
RNA, and protein has a remarkable capacity for adaptation to its
environment. We must learn more about body adaptability to
help maintain dynamic equilibria at optimal functioning without
yielding to the first stage of reversible disorganization accompanied by fatigue. We must continue to study the phenomenon
of fatigue in all its aspects—physical, mental, emotional and
sensual and define its parameters in terms of each individual
because there are times when the fate of man is not like a game
of chess dependent on skill, but like a lottery!

> *"Our stability is but balance, and wisdom lies*
> *in masterful administration of the unforeseen."*

I. Newton Kugelmass, M.D., Ph.D., Sc.D., *Editor*

Preface

THE PURPOSE OF THE BOOK IS TO KNIT TOGETHER SOME OF THE BEST UNDERSTANDING IN SEVERAL fields regarding a form of human inadequacy called fatigue. It is recognized that the human organism, though often dealt with in social terms is a biological system and must be treated as such if it is to be understood. While workers in a number of diverse fields have concerned themselves with what they call fatigue, there is a dearth of attempts to see the varied contributions in their proper light and to weave a single fabric out of them. It has been the purpose here to indicate the roles played by various orders of investigation, including chemistry, in building this understanding. If I have succeeded in providing something for readers to use in orienting themselves with regard to phenomenon as ubiquitous and as complex as fatigue, I shall feel gratified.

S. H. B.

Contents

FATIGUE

Mechanism and Management

CHAPTER ONE

Introduction

THE HUMAN ORGANISM LIVES IN A DEMANDING ENVIRONMENT. THE TYPES OF DEMAND ARE MANY and the ways the organism fails to meet these demands are also numerous. For example, these inadequacies include impairment, disorganization, frustration, fatigue, illness, etc. The diversity in possible states calls for a vocabulary and a language structure which recognizes all of them. Not only should they be recognized as entities but they should be defined in relation to each other. It is apparent that, for a long time, terminology and the thinking underlying it have not met this requirement. Fatigue, for example has become a word with vague, multiple and conflicting meanings. Its use ranges from reference to experienced discomfort in humans and their inability to do work, to reference to the inability of inanimate systems such as bridge girders to function normally.

This loose usage must be recognized as an impediment when setting out to deal with something called fatigue. At the outset the author must make clear what he is attempting to talk about when he uses the word, fatigue. This is best done by having reference to the class of phenomena in relation to other classes which are related but which are not to be called fatigue.

Such a clarification was made some years ago when Bartley and Chute wrote *Fatigue and Impairment in Man.* But this

3

does not obviate the need of a clarification prefacing a discussion of fatigue such as the present one.

The perseveration in using fatigue so variously and thus so loosely, is an expression of the more pervasive perseveration in the old non-biological way of viewing the human being. The trouble will remain until biology becomes effective enough to shift both the layman and the scientist into thinking and acting as though the human being were actually a biological system and its behavior fully describable and explainable in biological terms.

The subject of fatigue can well be dealt with by using an explicit set of selective principles. One can first ask, where and how was the word first used. Next he can ask whether the original reason for the usage still exists. And finally he may ask whether the added usages are natural extensions in the application of the term dictated by increase in human knowledge, or whether the new connotations have arisen simply by haphazard accretion; and therefore have brought about confusion rather than increased understanding.

It seems to be taken for granted that the extention in the use of words represents an evolution in understanding, but this is not always the case. Too much of the incidental and accidental often enters in and this has been the case with the use of the word fatigue.

It seems that the human, at least in certain societies, came to be able to discriminate among his feeling patterns and designate a condition called tiredness or fatigue. It was not always clear why he became tired but, in general, this feeling seemed to be associated with work and effort. The pervasive question, particularily when society reached the stage of taking human problems into the laboratory, became "What makes people tired?" It has been this ever since, though among laboratory workers, the problem has been broken into sub-problems, and the initial question has either been masked in various ways or entirely lost.

In what we shall have to say, we are returning to the original usage of the word and the original problem and are attempting to utilize the advances in scientific understanding that will bear upon it. Many of these advances are diverse and disconnected and have not yet been woven into cloth that can be used.

Definition of Fatigue. To begin with, fatigue did not have the many connotations that it now has been given. It referred only to how people felt in relation to some sort of activity. It thus had one meaning, the aversion toward activity and the feeling of inability to perform. This included experiences regarding the body and observations with regard to performance.

Fatigue was a self-recognized state of the individual. It was a directly experienced condition with an inferred connection between the way the individual felt and the amount he had exerted himself. Thus, the more work, the more tiredness. Quickly connections between fatigue and work output became closely associated. When fatigue was taken into the laboratory to be studied, decrement in work output became a synonymn and finally a definition for fatigue. This made fatigue not a condition of the worker, but a label for what he produced.

People in general, however, have continued to use their feelings and sensations to measure their capacity for activity and task achievement. The problem they still ask of the scientist is, "What makes people tired?"

It may be worthwhile at this point to classify the apparent views with regard to using the word, fatigue. (1) The first and broadest is that the word pertains to anything anybody wants it to. (2) It is a word, pertaining to biological systems only; but within such limits, it is a term applicable to all levels of description. That is, the person as a total can be tired, so can a muscle fiber, or a neuron. Fatigue is manifested by reduction performance. (3) Fatigue is a term applicable only in describing people, total organisms, not sub-systems or tissue within the organism.

This last alternative is in keeping with the original use of the term and is the alternative we are adopting. Our position is in line with the principle that each level of description should have its own vocabulary and language. This avoids anthropomorphisms and figures of speech, etc. which should have no place in science, where interrelation and causation are the chief things to be understood.

Several attempts have been made to eliminate the indiscriminate use of the word, fatigue. In 1921, Muscio (41), after having made an extensive study of tests for fatigue in humans, concluded that there was no single state that could be called fatigue or given any other single label, and suggested abandoning the term altogether. He suggested simply labelling each of the separate states or conditions by its own word. This, of course, was one logical possibility. But there is another, namely, the retention of the term fatigue for *one* of these states, and the use of other labels for the others. This is, in effect, the alternative just suggested.

Bartley (4, 7, 8, 9, 10, 11) and then Bartley and Chute (5, 6) and Gross and Bartley (22) took this way out. They chose the word's original meaning and defined fatigue as the sensory-cognitive syndrome which includes tiredness, aversion to work, body discomfort, ineffectiveness in performance, etc. This view implied that all that forestalls performance is not fatigue. The cause of work decrement might lie in local tissue and not be manifested as a personalistic syndrome. By personalistic is meant the organism acting as a whole (i.e., as a person). The term is somewhat of a substitute for the term, psychological. It is preferred because it doesn't retain the unfortunate dualistic connotation of referring to a mind as something different and apart from the body, but nevertheless, as something responsible for certain human activities. They suggested impairment as a term for cellular dysfunction illustrated, for example, in oxygen lack and various intoxications. This is an example of the principle already mentioned, namely, that of labelling phenomena in keeping with the organizational level of their biological involvement.

Even earlier, Whiting and English (60) had made a kind of distinction between fatigue and impairment by advancing the hypothesis that fatigue is a "negative emotional appetite," and that the psysiological phenomenon of exhaustion, is to be distinguished from it. They declared that fatigue was a "subjective" phenomenon. This, of course, may have had something to do with the failure of others to look unfavorably on their distinction, since anything declared to be "subjective" has long been set aside as unfit material for scientific investigation, at least in some disciplines.

In the present book we shall continue to limit the meaning of the term. We shall mean in general, what people originally meant when people said they were tired.

Fatigue then is an experienced self-evaluation. It is the aversion to activity, a condition of existence expressed in bodily feelings, a self-felt assessment of inadequacy, and the experience of futility, etc., with the desire to escape.

In this book we shall be faced with two problems. The one is to analyze fatigue and the conditions that produce it; the other, to deal with the management of fatigue as a symptom or a syndrome that is presented to the physician and others for alleviation.

Fatigue Performance, and Energy. Frequently fatigue has become confused with other conditions, including simply the inability to perform. When the ability to perform is actually the central concern it should be studied as such without pretending that it is fatigue.

Two apparent discrepancies show up under the attempt to interrelate fatigue and allied features. The first emerges in predictions about the ability to perform made from the physiological study of input-output relations in energistic terms. These predictions often do not tally with what the organism as a person is able to do. He comes to the quitting ("exhaustion") point before he fulfills the energistic prediction. This poses a puzzle about behavior causation.

The second discrepancy is the non-correspondence between performance and the way people feel. In some of the earlier experimental studies, it seemed that fatigue (as originally defined) and performance had little connection. This led to labelling the feeling, *subjective* fatigue, and decrement in work performance *objective* fatigue, with the result that "subjective" fatigue was generally laid aside as unworthy of investigation.

Fatigue as Dealt with Outside the Laboratory. Even when fatigue is used by individuals referring to themselves, there are two major ways this is done. In one case, individuals may be reporting upon how they feel. That is, they may be saying that they *feel* tired and unable to perform. Or, in the other case, they may be using the word fatigue as a label for an *inference*. They note certain things about themselves and *conclude* that these are signs of fatigue. In this case they are, in effect, making a diagnosis and are not reporting directly on tired feelings at all. What is being referred to in the two cases is vastly different, and cannot be dealt with in the same way.

It is difficult to tell just how many different items may be used as the basis for the self-diagnosis. Any physician accepting this self-diagnosis is led astray. In our outlook on the matter, this use of the term is to be excluded even though whatever it may be that leads to using the term fatigue may lie in the realm of inadequacy, personalistically defined.

Even when we confine ourselves to the cases in which tired-ness refers to how the individual feels and evaluates himself, the cases are not all strictly alike. In some cases, the individual is satiated with the events or conditions around him. He is "fed up," bored or annoyed. He does not feel able to endure any more of the same. He may be in a situation in which no particular positive action or accomplishment (work product) is required, but nevertheless existence is unpleasant and escape seems to be the only thing that will provide recovery.

In other cases, tiredness accrues from something different. An intellectual achievement is required or being attempted. A point is reached in which progress is slowed, or achievement seems impossible. In this situation, like the previous one, no great energistic exertion is involved at all. It is not a question of possessing a metabolism that will maintain muscular activity at a high rate. Nevertheless, the individual feels he cannot go on. His thinking becomes disorganized and to the extent that he is aware of this he becomes tired. In common parlance this is called mental fatigue. But if such a term is to be retained, the implication that mental fatigue is essentially any different than any other kind should be discarded. We would simply say that this fatigue is the fatigue that arises in an intellectual task, rather than implying that it is essentially different than other fatigues.

A third type of situation in which tiredness arises is the exertional task. Here the crucial factor is the maintenance of muscular activity at a given level. This activity has various bodily consequences which slow down work output and thus conflicts with the performer's purposes. At the same time the individual begins to feel bodily uncomfortable. It is difficult, if at all possible, here to dissociate the direct bodily feeling consequent to prolonged muscular activity from the personalistic component, the feeling of inadequacy as a performer of the task at hand. Obviously those who study behavior under exertional conditions have something quite tangible to investigate and to concentrate upon. Here the various facets of metabolism become the objects of study. Here fatigue and reduced effectiveness of body machinery become synonymous in the thinking of the investigators.

The point that we want to make is that in each of the three widely different types of situations, it is the human individual, the organism-as-a-person that is aware of his inadequacy. It is this feeling of inability to carry on that is the core of the matter and it is this that is essentially the fatigue. The "trimmings" are different but the essential stance or relation of the organism to the environment is the same. It is this common core that allows us to call all the varieties of the syndrome by a single name, fatigue. It is this that Muscio did not deal with in the varities of conditions which he studied. The tests he used were tests for different *kinds* of achievement, hence it is no wonder that they did not tally with each other. Since they didn't, he came to the conclusion he was dealing with a variety of largely unrelated phenomena. He was correct about sheer differences of achievement, but had he been dealing with the nature of the organism's relation to the environment, he could have seen an essential similarity in the variety.

It has always been difficult for investigators and theorists to isolate this common denominator from the obstrusive variety of phenomena manifested. It has been eluding investigators for a long time. The existence of this common stance or relation to the environment (to demand) is the very thing the reader should never lose sight of.

To summarize, it may be said that instead of using fatigue as a single or loose catch-all term, we had better recognize the envolvement of a group of quite distinguishable elements in the total situation. They are impairment, disorganization, discomfort, largely localized in muscles, work decrement, and finally fatigue.

Impairment is the reduced ability of the cells to function. Disorganization is modification in the ways of cells, tissues and organs working together. This may happen, at least in the nervous system without impairment, for it is one of the chief properties of the nervous system to be able to manifest all kinds of organizational variation. For example, all that one need do to change nervous function and its consequences, is to tell a performer that he is failing. This sensory input changes the whole pattern of nervous function, without initially impairing cells. As a consequence not only nervous function but muscular function becomes disorganized. This does not mean wholesale disintegration, as is often the connotation of the word, but simply a change in organization less appropriate for achieving the given ends. Awkwardness is an example of disorganization. Skill is an example of appropriate organization. Discomfort arises through sensory mechanisms being effected by tissue changes including those called impairment. Work decrement is the measurable drop in activity of muscles measured in energistic terms, or the drop in intellectual productivity measured in other terms. Both of these decrements may be externally measured in units of production. Fatigue is the individual's assessment of his condition with reference to his immediate task. It is an overall appraisal expressed in bodily feelings, and the realization of reduced effectiveness, etc.

For many years now, those studying the inability of individuals to perform have been focussing on impairment while calling it and the other components, fatigue. This view has taken for granted that once what we have called impairment is understood and controlled, the total problem will be solved. How the organism as a person functions has been called an epiphenomenon and bypassed as insignificant. Only the clinicians, and perhaps people in industry and sports have been faced with dealing with organisms as people, and thus have had to try to find ways of coping with what we call fatigue.

Fatigue as the Clinician Sees It. Various medical writers point out that fatigue and the feeling of energy lack are among the commonest complaints that they hear. Hence *chronic* fatigue is of predominant interest (2).

Harms and Soniat (23) list the following causes of the fatigue complaint. The first of these is dehibilitating illness. It is during the long convalescence from such illness that fatigue shows up in many patients. Here, the constitutional differences in people are at work. In our society, it is the person with initiative (the aggressive person) that is considered normal, the less active are given various labels that are not too complimentary. It is usually the less sturdy person who says he is fatigued, and on this account, these authors say that it is well to attempt to discover how much exertion such a person can tolerate. He must be taken as his own standard.

Harms and Soniat continue the listing of causes of fatigue as lack of motivation, nervous tension and anxiety, depression, hysteria, chronic inhibition of ego function. These do not seem to be expressions apart from the individual's value system just mentioned.

Snow, Machlan, Warnell and Utt (55) also indicate that the number of patients who seek medical help for chronic fatigue is "legion." The main complaint of this group of patients is "undue fatigability, mild depression, and chronic constipation." Frequently they complain of aches and stiffness in joints, but show no organic changes. They often present signs such as dry skin, brittle nails, muscle tenderness and menstrual irregularities. For such patients, the typical treatment is thyroid extract, the amphetamines, barbituates, and tranquilizers, all of which these authors say produce unsatisfactory results. Adrenocortical insufficiency and vitamin deficiency have been supposed to underlie the fatigue, but neither corticosteroid nor vitamin therapy have proved to be of satisfactory benefit, they say.

Nussbaum (43) reminds us that fatigue patients fall into two classes, the organically tired individual who is exhausted by very little effort, and the psychogenically tired person who becomes tired from merely anticipating effort. This individual is often benefited by the very activity that tires the organically insufficient. This distinction is quite reminiscent of Muncie's (40) earlier classification.

Friedlander (19) classifies the psychogenically fatigue patients into: (1) those with simple reactive anxiety and depression, patients presenting an immediate history of traumatic experience; (2) those with exhaustive depression which he calls "managerial disease"; since they are common among executives and those undergoing "intellectual distress"; (3) those with neurotic anxiety and depression in which there is complaint of isolation and helplessness in connection with the tiredness; (4) those with involutional depressions, effecting both males and females, at senescent and menopausal periods respectively; and (5) those with the endogenous depression, complaining of despondency rather than fatigue, although the complaint is interpreted by the patient as fatigue. Variations in this spectrum present themselves, but it is up to the diagnostic perceptiveness of the physician to successfully identify the pattern he finds.

These authors state that an unfortunate record of ineffective attempts at relief and cure has characterized the history of fatigue. This has been the basis for their trying new procedures and new substances.

The Role of Chemistry and Metabolism in Fatigue. The question of the role body chemistry plays in the production and alleviation of fatigue turns out to be a very pressing problem in the common outlook on fatigue for certainly it makes a vast difference as to whether the difficulty is something that can be treated by correcting or boosting body process, or whether the remedy is one of changing the organism as a person. The present book is cognizant of the relevance of the very old question, namely, *what avenues* can be used to beneficially influence human condition and human behavior. It involves answering the question of what circumstances call for dealing with the individual as a *person* who can be influenced through his senses, etc., through effects upon his thought processes; and what circumstances call for dealing with the individual through other avenues, such as the administration of drugs or through altering the basic physical demands.

Whom Is This Analysis For? One may ask who needs to understand the analysis of fatigue as it is being presented here. Obviously this analysis is made for the sophisticated worker in the field of human inadequacy. It is firmly belived that research on fatigue can not progress while there is no clear understanding of the distinction between phenomena at various levels ranging from sheer biochemistry to perception and cognition in the individual. Fatigue has too long been used as a loose group label for unknown causes of reduced performance and inability. Pointing out the difference between fatigue, impairment, etc., should certainly aid the investigator.

The analysis should help the physician. Among other things, he must be aware of the differences between using fatigue as a label for miscellaneous symptoms of inadequacy supplied either by himself or by the patient, and the use of fatigue as a label by the patient for his own *directly felt* inadequacy and task aversion.

The athletic coach, also should participate in this clarification of fatigue and other features of inadequacy. It should enable him to know better what to expect of his trainees and contestants than otherwise.

All of the persons just mentioned might well be expected to comprehend that the organism is a unitary system wherein body process accounts for all known varieties of phenomena pertaining to the human, be they phenomena of metabolism, or be they phenomena which are cognitive. The age-old implication that cognitive (mental) phenomena are apart from body process should be discarded.

Perhaps little can be expected of the public at present. Its insights and understandings await the rectification in the thinking and vocabularies of the classes of persons just mentioned, in the direction suggested, whereby an example is given for public thinking and understanding to follow.

It is hoped that this brief resume of the distinction between fatigue, impairment, work output, and assayed energistic resources of the individual has provided a clarification, and will form an orientation for considering the material in subsequent chapters.

In the chapters that follow, the topic of fatigue will be dealt with under the following major headings: (1) fatigue situations; (2) forms of inadequacy contributing to fatigue; (3) the mechanism of fatigue; (4) the role of body chemistry in fatigue and inadequacy; (5) prevalent pharmaceutical agents used to combat fatigue and inadequacy; and finally (6) some remarks on the management of fatigue.

CHAPTER TWO

Fatigue Situations

FATIGUE IS A CONDITION OF THE INDIVIDUAL AND IS NOT TO BE DEFINED IN TERMS OF EXTERNAL SITUA-tions or even work products. Nevertheless some situations in which people find themselves are typically fatigue-producing. It would be profitable, in coming to a better understanding of fatigue itself, to examine these situations to see what it is that they demand of the individual. All situations that are relevant to our discussion make demands on the individual. We need to know what kinds of demands are typically made.

The Expenditure of Energy. The first class of fatigue-producing situations consists of those that require considerable expenditures of energy. It is this class of situations that has received, by far, the most study. In fact, it is from this type of study and from concepts associated with it that most of the prevalent notions of fatigue have emerged. The question has usually been, how much work can an individual perform and what are the effects upon the person who performs it. This has meant, how good an energy utilizer or transformer is the human organism. Various conditions are set up to test this, and measuring input-output relations has received a great deal of study. Precise studies of this sort done in laboratories of physiology, biochemistry and nutrition have yielded much important knowledge (17, 18).

In such studies, the question of how the performer feels

may or may not be considered. Most often this question is entirely omitted, of course, the reason for this being that feelings are not "objective," or that no way of quantifying them has been discovered, or that they do not relate to the ability to perform work.

Quite typically, the terminal conditions of performance, often called exhaustion, are ascertained. The concept of fatigue involved belongs to class 2 in the classification presented in the preceeding chapter. "Fatigue" generally turns out to be something measured in reduced worn output. As we see it, such studies are examples of ascertaining productivity rather than of ascertaining either how the worker feels or what the cost to the worker is. For our purposes *work output* as such, and the *condition* of the worker are to be distinguished as separate entities.

What is there about energy-expending tasks that pertains to fatigue as we define it? It has long been recognized that expending energy produces effects in the expender. These effects occur at various levels of organization within the individual. Some of them are metabolic, some are sensory, and some are the results of learning. Metabolic changes in addition to energistic incapacitation for work, lead to sensory discomfort, and at the cognitive level, these symptoms are the fuel for the individual's aversion to continuing performance.

The task of anyone studying the results of exertion on the performer leading to fatigue is to trace the changes in process which limit overt performance, how discomfort is produced, how this yields the eventual inability of the organism as a person to carry on.

Exertional performance is often of either one or the other of two patterns. Either the performance produces enough sensory discomfort that the individual stops before he has reached what might be called the physiological limit, or else he dashes into heavy exertion and in some respects "over does" it before he becomes aware of it. Only later does he find that he has been quite injudicious. This is particularly true of older sedentary individuals, who often seem able to perform some task to which they are unaccustomed and only later discover the price they have paid. The results brought about in the activity of the physically "trained" and hardened individual are undoubtedly of the first sort. Such individuals may experience considerable tiredness without suffering subsequent ill consequences.

Paced Performance. A second class of situations which typically produces fatigue consists in those demands that pace or otherwise restrict the individual's performance. We must always consider the degree of freedom or degree of restrictedness imposed upon the performer by external conditions when we want to understand the cost of any activity to him. The individual left to himself, tends to do things his own way and at his own speed. Even when many of his acts are sterotyped by habit they are free from the imposition of formal demands. To the extent that activity is inherently determined within the performer himself, it can continue great lengths of time. To the extent that the way acts are to be performed or how fast they are to be performed, are externally determined there is likely to be a conflict between demand and the manner in which the acts tend to be performed. There is often considerable discrepancy between the two. The worker subjecting himself to externally imposed requirements, is demanding of himself a more difficult order of organization within the neuromuscular system than when free to manifest variety, randomness of movement, or even when his habituated activity has the outward appearance of being constrained.

Many tasks that people are called upon to perform involve what we would describe as pacing. The feeding of a machine, or the retrieval of material from a machine at a given rate and a given way are good examples of pacing. Perhaps when pacing involves simple enough movements, the performance is like marching or dancing. It can be done with ease and enjoyment. Many tasks that involve pacing, or other restrictedness are not that simple nor that enjoyable. Writing is a good example. One must form the letters and words on the page according to certain rules, in order that they be legible. The writer cannot make just any movement that he tends to. Furthermore there is a timing discrepancy between the speed of thinking and the speed of writing. The urge to hurry to keep up with thinking often results in a gradual deterioration in penmanship and writing progress. This deterioration is an outward manifestation of the development of neuromuscular disorganization. The individual gradually uses more and more widespread, and thus more redundant, musculature as he goes along. His hand gets tense; his arm gets tense. The tenseness finally pervades his whole body. Eventually this condition becomes the basis for the attitudinal and sensory complex we call fatigue.

Reading tasks are also good examples of restricted performances. Eye movements in such situations cannot be of the free wandering sort characteristic of idle, random vision.

Various other tasks required in everyday life are of the paced or restricted type, and for this reason if for no other, they form the basis for disorganization of process and eventual fatigue.

Prolonged Activity. The crucial features of some tasks is the length of time they require. They might never produce fatigue were they less prolonged. The prolongation is a form of restrictedness. This, in a way, relates such tasks to those we have just described. Both types produce the same end results, disorganization of process, bodily discomfort, reduced output and eventual fatigue, the performer's sensory-cognitive evaluation of inability to meet demand.

Action in the Face of Remoteness of Goals. Fatigue has been found to develop quite quickly in tasks in which the goals are quite remote. In such cases various negative features associated with the activity stand out sometimes as relatively more effective than the goals themselves and fatigue sets in, not as a result of energy expenditure but from the general attitude occuring from the remoteness of the goal to be achieved.

Frustrating Situations. Some situations in which performance and accomplishment are attempted may truly be frustrating. While frustration, as we define it, is a state of the individual and not a characteristic of an external situation, some situations are much more likely to produce frustrations. Thus while we call them frustrating situations, the frustration is not something descriptive of the situations themselves.

What kinds of situations would produce frustration? Among those most likely to do this would be those which involve conflicting performance requirements, or possess conflicting features in other respects. Conflicts can be inherent in the specified demands from the very start, or conflicts can develop through changes in demands, wherein one kind of performance is required at one time, and other kinds at other times, with no forewarning, or without any obvious rationale for the changes. Frustration is the state the individual is put into by such conditions. A cognitive aspect of this state is the performer's realization that continuing performance is largely futile. In the situations of this general class, the performer may find his way blocked regardless of which way he turns. He finds that what he is able to accomplish is slight and has no relation to the ingenuity or effort he applies. This is bound to reflect not only in lack of work accomplished but in the psychophysiology of the performer. The results are describable in body process terms as well as in feelings. The salient end-result in terms of the performer's experience is fatigue. Although this be the case, he is often puzzled as to why this has occurred. This puzzlement stems, of course, from the prevalent tacit assumption that fatigue is an outcome only of energy expenditure and that energy expenditure and work output should tally. Since little muscular effort may have been involved in the situation in question, little fatigue should have ensued. In fact the puzzlement itself may be a contributor to further fatigue. Situations in which goals are unclear, often turn out to be frustration-producing situations.

Limiting Conditions. Various external circumstances impose demands which involve considerable difficulty for the human organism to meet, or which, in existing, modify basic biological function. These factors are well called *limiting conditions*. The major examples of limiting conditions are oxygen, water and salt and sugar deprivation, and temperature extremes. It is easy to see that these and other such factors limit behavior. In so doing they lead to deteriorative performance and thus may preclude the carrying out of purpose. Some limiting conditions may involve the operation of the nervous system in ways so as to eliminate the self-critical ability of the performer. When the self-evaluation ability of the performer is reduced fatigue may be precluded although impairment may be extreme, and overt accomplishment be reduced to nothing. Cases of this sort are much like cases of alcoholic intoxication. In both the performer's evaluation of his own behavior becomes blunted or distorted.

In certain circumstances limiting conditions may operate to preclude or reduce performance while not impairing the performer's self-awareness and self-evaluation. In such cases fatigue does ensue. Such cases are good examples to illustrate the ultimate dependence of fatigue upon self-evaluation rather than merely upon reduced performance or failure of accomplishment.

While oxygen deprivation is not frequently a characteristic of every day living situations, it is an example of one of the more effective kinds of limiting conditions. It occurs for some in high altitudes. In earlier years of aviation, it was a major factor that was not effectively taken care of. It is a major factor to conjure with in mountain climbing.

Oxygen lack can be involved, not through its absence in the air that is breathed but through inadequate functioning of tissues within the organism: In certain illnesses, extra oxygen must be supplied to compensate for such difficulties. Oxygen lack is a problem in anemia.

In all cases in which the deprivation is considerable, but not so sudden or so extreme as to induce the individual's inability to be aware of the malfunctioning manifested in overt performance of insensory loss or distortion, oxygen lack tends to contribute to fatigue.

Water lack, while not necessarily very closely tied to classes of work situations, is probably more common than supposed. Actual thirst is no good criterion, in man, for determining water intake. Some dehydration can exist without the individual experiencing thirst. Some degree of water deficiency is a greater possibility among people than is generally recognized. While definite dehydration does produce symptoms, lesser and generally not recognized symptoms are brought about by borderline circumstances. Some of these symptoms include vague discomfort which can be an underlying factor in developing a distaste for job activity. When prolonged this becomes a definite contributor to fatigue (weariness and tiredness).

The common low spells in mid morning and mid afternoon may involve sugar lack, in low blood sugar levels. Eating and drinking at these times are known to alleviate symptoms. How much this becomes an individual or a social habit is hard to say. It has been shown that distribution of food intake does hold blood sugar levels up for greater percentages of the total work day than where meals are fewer. The precise nature of the interrelations between coffee breaks, blood sugar level and the feelings of tiredness etc., have not yet been fully worked out. Haggard and Greenberg, for example, a few years ago made a good start.

It is possible that the metabolic processes of individuals become conditioned to diurnal patterns of water and food intake, so that blood sugar levels and water loads of some people may have characteristics not typical of people in other occupations where replenishment is not so frequent and yet in which not untoward symptomatology is evident.

For several sorts of reason, then, it would not be surprising if individuals used to mid morning or mid afternoon breaks would get tired and become less effective when the breaks are not available.

High temperature coupled with exertion may reduce salt concentration through sweating, to the point of producing incapacitation for further exertion. This matter, too, is somewhat complicated, and no simple cause and effect description is adequate. The relation between chloride levels, work capacity, and fatigue is, nevertheless, a matter not to be overlooked.

To say the least, the affect of limiting conditions is varied and complex and they are not too concretely discernible by the performer himself. The only thing he knows real well is that he gets tired and weary. Why, is not too clear. The types of deprivation (limiting conditions) has possible significant factors.

Demand Too Exacting for a Specific Body Mechanism. In this class of situations it is not certain whether we are dealing with matters best handled in this chapter or in the following one in which forms of inadequacy of the performer himself contribute mainly to fatigue. We can at least, introduce the problem in this chapter, even though it may also be relevant later.

Some task demands focus primarily upon what some particular body mechanism is required to do. This is particularly true in the case of the senses, vision in particular,

While our culture has greatly reduced simple exertional demands on muscle, it has also increased the complex and exacting forms of interaction with the environment. Such demands are best exemplified in vision where body mechanisms are required to relate in a very precise and complex way with external circumstances.

Vision is both motor and sensory. It is accomplished by certain reflexes coordinating these two factors. In fact there are several motor components to effective vision. The two eyes must be converged on the visual target, they must be moved in proper coordination when looking about or when the target moves, and the focusing mechanism (accommodation), handled by the change in the thickness of the lens must be coordinated with target distance and the muscular process just mentioned. While this matter is essentially a reflex affair and possesses certain involuntary and inherent characteristics that are not directly controlled by the knowledge and wishes of the performer, visual behavior, to some extent, can be modified. Part of the development of the individual in the ability to see is to be understood as habit formation. All achievements of this kind are open to some distortion and ineffectiveness.

Vision is also based upon structural factors (the anatomy, the eyes, etc.). These have long been the center of attention both in the science of vision, and in the professional practice of eye care. It has become evident that all individuals are not equally able to carry on certain visual tasks (reading, etc.) that our society demands.

Fatigue frequently does arise from visual work. It should not be called visual fatigue in the common usage of the term. The fatigue produced is the same personalistic phenomenon that is produced when other situations make people tired. It is only visual in the sense that, visual performance has occasioned it.

The literal symptoms that occur may be headache, blurring, diplopia, lachrimation, tensions around the eyes, etc. What is frequently called fatigue then is simply an inference that these symptoms must bespeak of some vague underlying thing that one should call fatigue. This is in contrast to the actual tiredness produced by trying to perform the visual task, the actual direct sensory-cognitive outcome that we call fatigue.

Conditions for Chronic Fatigue. The final description of untoward situations is not made until one includes chronic fatigue. Here, of all places, the question of what causes fatigue becomes most subtle. Fatigue that crops up day after day, or continues over long periods, perhaps involves little that can be put into terms as specific as already mentioned. It would seem here we are dealing with a "way fo life."

While chronic fatigue may be looked upon from the standpoint of some deficiency in the individual in question, such fatigue can arise from conditions that lie in the environment. It is this that we have reference to here. Some environments are such as to produce fatigue in the vast majority of people. They include a great many things that can be classed as frustration, or as futile and therefore they lead to a chronic stance which has as its chief characteristic the feeling of inability, weakness, and tiredness. The remedy may lay in changing the environment or in the far more unlikely thing, namely changing the whole fundamental life philosophy of the individual.

Conclusions

It should be clear from what has been said so far that our concern in discussing and/or dealing with fatigue is of three sorts. The first has to do with the effects of exertion. This is to say we need to know what happens in the body as a result of expending energy. Most of the energy transformation takes place in muscle, hence a great deal of attention is to be paid to what goes on in muscle.

The second class of phenomenon that concerns us is the organization of processes within the body. Organization is something that occurs at various levels. Much of it is neuromuscular and is involved in performing acts of skill or meeting demands in which activity is of a restricted or predetermined form. To understand how fatigue develops in such situations is to understand matters relating to the *organization* of internal activity rather than to *energy expenditure.*

The third concern has to do with the relation of the organism as a person to the environment.

CHAPTER THREE

Forms of Inadequacy Contributing to Fatigue

A NUMBER OF CHRONIC ANOMALOUS CONDITIONS, EVEN IF MILD, MAY CONTRIBUTE TO THE DEVELOPment of fatigue. A few of these will be dealt with in this chapter. No attempt will be made to mention all of them. Those mentioned simply serve as major illustrations of the fact that bodily dysfunctions may incapacitate the individual for exertion and/or for sustained attention to intellectual tasks and therefore underlie task aversion and what we call fatigue.

Hypothyroidism (Myxedema). This condition, an inadequacy of the thyroid gland presents various symptoms such as low basal metabolism, inability to keep awake, marked intolerance for cold, slowness of thought and action, muscle weakness and backache, among others. While these symptoms may not all be severe, they obviously relate to task performance and accomplishment. They are certainly conditions which would tend to make the individual inadequate for many kinds of tasks and even ineffective in general every day affairs. To the extent that this is apparent to the individual, he would tire easily. He would possess the feelings and self-evalution we call fatigue.

Hypochondria. Hypochondria is characterized by a state of extreme concern regarding bodily health and the proper functioning of the various bodily organs. The hypochondriac is preoccupied with himself and how he feels. (Individuals with hypochondria become vividly aware of all kinds of minor bodily changes and sensations of no significance in themselves but which they interpret as serious.) He is keenly related to the circumstances around him through his feelings. From this it is easy to see that certain kinds of demands would be more effective in producing states of negative self-evaluation than in the case of normals. He would be more likely to have the idea that continued activity is hurtful and thus develop task-aversion symptomatology earlier than other people. Hence the hypochondriac is a prime candidate for fatigue.

Neurasthenia, Psychasthenia. Some individuals in which no definite picture of organ disease can be identified, seem to be unable to carry on much exertion and are quite irritable. Events which ordinarily are taken to be quite minor may produce quite marked irritation and bodily consequences. These states somewhat resemble certain anxiety states, except that feelings of apprehension and intense anxiety are missing. The experience of weakness appears after little effort of any sort, be it physical or intellectual.

This is asthenia and is characterized by headaches, backaches, pain in the extremities, gastrointestinal disturbances, blurring after short periods of reading, loss of libido, and frigidity.

When inadequacy is associated mainly with bodily activity, the term neurasthenia is often applied. When the effect is mostly expressed in intellectual sluggishness, inability to concentrate, etc., the term psychasthenia is often used.

It is obvious that such individuals manifest a picture of general inadequacy, and fatigue is one of the chief ways this is expressed.

Effort Syndrome. Effort syndrome is but one of several labels for a syndrome which has been described by various writers. The other names are neurocirculatory asthenia, Da Costas' syndrome, irritable heart, disordered action of the heart, soldiers' heart, and anxiety neurosis. It is possible that those who write on this subject are not all actually describing the very same syndrome, although the descriptions possess considerable in common. As might be expected, the designations either seize upon a single prominent feature of the syndrome or reflect what the writer of the given report believes to be a primary factor in its etiology.

"Irritable heart" was detected in the Crimean War. In the American Civil War, Da Costa (16) studied 300 cases of cardiac difficulty. The trouble he found showed up after the soldier was in service for some time. Two-thirds of the cases were between sixteen and twenty-five years of age. The first symptom was frequently diarrhea. Rapid pulse was another, and this outlasted the gastrointestinal trouble. The symptoms summarized by Da Costa were: (1) palpitation, most readily induced by exertion; (2) "cardiac pain"; (3) shortness of breath and oppression on exertion; (4) rapid pulse; (5) headaches, giddiness, disturbed sleep, itching skin and excessive perspiration; and (6) indigestion, abdominal distension and diarrhea. When the individual was returned to duty he could not seem to keep up with his comrades.

Da Costa saw the difficulty as a somatic affair, due to heavy duty and hardships. He saw the trouble stemming from a heart that had become irritable from overactivity and had been sustained in this condition by disordered innervation. Improvement in general health did not fully relieve the trouble.

During the First World War, cases such as already described, again began to show up frequently. A distinction was made between cases involving true organic inadequacy and those that were but a part of a larger pattern of disorder. Sir Thomas Lewis (33) listed the characteristics of the latter type of cases. The label now became "effort syndrome." The symptoms were: (1) breathlessness, cyanosis slight or absent; (2) pain; (3) palpitation; (4) fainting; (5) giddiness; (6) headaches after exertion; (7) complaints of fatigue.

Civilian cases have also been reported. These differed in one respect at least. Dyspnea and rapid breathing persisted during sleep, whereas they did not in the military cases. In Lewis' cases, the most common type of breathlessness was in connection with exertion. Lewis stressed the complaint of fatigue, having found it almost without exception. In keeping with this symptom, the posture drooped and the face was pallid. There was hand tremor and unsteadiness in the legs. Lewis concluded from case histories that infection was a common factor lying behind these cases. The term neurocirculatory asthenia was suggested by the British. Later the psychogenic origin of the syndrome was recognized and stressed. Robey and Boas (46) stressed "fundamental nervous instability" as a basic factor in neurocirculatory asthenia. Others still attributed the trouble to something basically wrong with the heart. Some state that the type of electrocardiogram obtained from patients with the syndrome show that such patients have small and underdeveloped hearts.

In direct contrast to this, other writers have suggested hyperventilation as a causative factor. Actual hyperventilation does lead to a set of consequences known as the hyperventilation syndrome. Accordingly some writers have suggested diagnosing the condition as an anxiety state complicated by the hyperventilation syndrome.

Nowadays, the effort syndrome is seen as a definitely psychomatic disorder and the psychogenic origin is recognized. The emotional reaction arises from a misinterpretation of the symptoms resulting from effort. It is said that the overall pattern stems from such factors as: (1) family background; (2) constitutional timidity; (3) bodily symptoms such as breathlessness, fatigue, palpitation, etc.; (4) and certain deeper lying physical signs.

Immerman (27) suggests dividing the effort syndrome patients into two groups: (1) the asthenic, and (2) the neurorespiratory. Wittkower and colleagues (62) made a five class division of their cases: (1) patients with keen sense of duty and not wishing to show fear; (2) resigned grousers, with insubordination and poor interpersonal relations; (3) overaggressive rebels; (4) those with inferior physiques and obsessive drives to compensate; (5) hysterical quitters. Certain writers agree fairly well with this classification.

For our purpose we need simply to recognize that there is a type of individual who, for some reason, has shown bodily symptoms in connection with effort and has come to interpret these as significant and as signs of danger. We might actually say that this syndrome has some characteristics of hypochrondriasis, a kind expressed in specific conditioned (learned) patterns of response to demand for exertion.

Postural Hypotension. The inability to stand long or walk distances without exhaustion or collapse is a known clinical entity. It is sometimes called orthostatic hypotension and is characterized by the following: (1) failure of the pulse rate to rise when the subject rises to a standing position; (2) diminition or absence of sweating; (3) loss of sexual desire; (4) pallor; (5) high blood urea; (6) low basal metabolism.

Despite the clarity of the hypotension symptoms, the physician sometimes finds it difficult to relate them to a broader set of conditions. That is, he is unable to discover the origin of the difficulty. It is entirely possible that, in some cases at least, habit formation (conditioning) is responsible. In such cases, the symptoms seem to have a meaningful connection to the cognitive affairs of the individual.

The following example possibly illustrates that conditioning is a factor. Various men report becoming extremely tired and exhausted from shopping with their wives. A great part of this shopping from the man's standpoint consists in standing around while waiting for his wife to browse and to make purchases. There is nothing in particular for the husband to do and he often finds himself in the way of the customers around him. Some men have been known to feel as though they would collapse. One man, in slight panic asked for a chair, to keep from collapsing. This individual was not particularly inadequate in various other situations. He was accustomed to playing tennis quite regularly. Whatever label can be put upon this particular case, the man is only one of many who feel quite inadequate, weak, tired and subject to headaches in shopping situations. Whether the feelings of weakness, exhaustion etc., are accompanied by measurable symptoms of organ dysfunction such as hypotension and allied symptoms is not definitely known. From the psychic standpoint the matter has all the appearance of a conditioned response. It is known that some victims of this difficulty produced in shopping situations do not have a similar reaction when they wait on the sidewalk for their wives or others to meet them.

It is possible that there is some connection between the type of case just described and the clinical cases of postural hypotension, by way of both being, in part, conditioned responses.

To say the least, proneness to symptoms of the sort described is a basis for fatigue.

Myasthenia Gravis. This is a chronic disease in which the muscles are very easily made inactive by little exertion. While this affliction is not too common it does occur in mild forms and is usually of gradual onset. It is thought the trouble is induced at the myoneural junction by the excessive action of cholinesterase upon acetylcholine. Prostigmine and similar drugs are given to combat this by lowering the level of cholinesterase in the blood. Muscular incapacitation that is involved in this disease can easily lead to fatigue through the feeling of inability and futility that is engendered.

Arthritis and Rheumatism. These painful afflictions of the joints and muscles disenable motor activity. Those who find themselves victims of this type of incapacity are also among the most likely candidates for fatigue.

Emphysema. This disease is symptomatized by a number of features, the prime one being dyspnea. Although this may be somewhat periodic in its appearance, it emerges to incapacitate the individual quite severely at times. It is the kind of a difficulty that not only inactivates the individual when present, but may prove a conditioning factor in making persons wary of exertional activity in general, and thus easily fatigable.

Diabetes. This affliction exists in various degrees of severity from the very mild to the very severe. In some cases it is not recognized by the individual having it, perhaps both because it is mild and because he is not in the habit of having periodic physical examinations which might have disclosed it.

Whereas in severe cases there are very noticeable symptoms such as loss of weight, loss of strength, extremes of appetite, etc., in mild cases, these symptoms are absent in noticeable amounts. There is little or no loss of strength, and the discovery of the disease is only accidental or incidental to a check-up for some other reason.

Nevertheless, such a condition as diabetes is a likely basis for the individual's detecting his inadequacy in certain kinds of tasks, particularly those involving considerable exertion or those which are not particularly pleasant. While fatigue will arise in anyone when task situations are obnoxious, it may show up more readily in individuals with metabolic deficiencies, such as diabetes.

Depression. Depression is a background out of which definite complaints of fatigue may develop. It is for this reason that depression is listed here along with the more specific afflictions. At times, depression is simply considered a state that is associated with fatigue, with no attempt to indicate which is causal to the other. But here we are supposing that depression is an underlying factor in fatigue. According to some writers, 85 per cent of all the patients seen in private practice manifest chronic mild depression of some sort or other, this being associated with easy fatigability, frequent headaches, etc. Thus we have here a general picture, with several common symptoms and varied with a number of others. An examination of the literature on the forms of treatment of depressed states definitely shows that such patients actually differ quite markedly from each other and cannot all be treated the same way. This is borne out by the results obtained by the use of the various new drugs ranging from certain of the tranquilizers, to the so-called psychic energizers.

Depression, as it relates to fatigue, is a condition which, to say the least, is one in which medication may be of help. It is often very difficult to determine how the depressed state has arisen, whether as a by-product of an illness or a low grade under-par chronic condition or whether from some untoward and seemingly insoluable set of social circumstances encountered by the individual.

Medicine and psychology are coming more and more surely and clearly to see that many of the conventional distinctions made between body and mental conditions are not valid. Depression states often involve enough malfunction in body process to make them clinical entities which can, to a large extent, be attacked by medication. A careful examination of the patients condition will disclose some clues to what form of medication to attempt. However, success in the use of a drug or course of medication need not imply that the patient's difficulty is solely a matter which medication is alone responsible for alleviating. There are always two components to the affair. One is the body-process malfunction at the level of an organ system, and the interpretive process that occurs at a higher physiological level in the individual. If medication improves body process, it tends to improve body feeling. This is of at least temporary relief. The patient's interpretation may be favorable and this adds to the relief. If certain bad habits of hygiene, or unfortunate ways the patient has of looking at daily routine and responsibilities underlie the depression, a reliance on medication as a total cure may bring disappointment. The medication which helps for a time finally loses its effectiveness.

In most, if not all cases, there is an unrecognized habit component in the patient's difficulty. He is in his condition as a result of the habits he has formed over long periods of time. The habits referred to here are those expressed as ways of reacting to the various little daily confrontations. The patient has come to dislike too many things that he confronts from day to day. Instead of developing a philosophy in which these items can become of much less consequence, he carries on an internal battle against them. Some people carry on this battle by voicing a talkative opposition. Others may remain quite silent, but in both cases, the battle goes on and is expressed by organ dysfunction of some sort or other. Medication provides boosters but in time the boosters of body function may fail. In later life we simply call this aging, and resign ourselves to such labels.

A great deal of preventative medicine will someday consist in proper habit formation.

Conclusions

In this chapter some of the many clinical syndromes that form the basis of personal inadequacy and fatigue have been briefly mentioned. The examples have been meant to indicate that the result we call fatigue can arise from something deficient in the individual as well as in something taxing about a task performance. In some cases these deficiencies are so great that the individual does not expect to do much. Other people do not expect much from him under such circumstances and he resigns himself to his condition. In other cases, the deficiency is much less and he expects as much of himself as if the deficiency did not exist. This discrepancy between aspiration and ability to accomplish becomes a significant thing in his daily life. The awareness is largely expressed in the feeling of fatigue. The individual should use himself as his own standard of what he should accomplish, rather than to set his goal by some external standard and constantly find he cannot reach it.

CHAPTER FOUR

The Mechanisms Underlying Fatigue

THE PURPOSE OF THIS CHAPTER IS TO DESCRIBE THE MECHANISMS OF FATIGUE. THIS CONSISTS IN DEALING with what goes on in the individual and what occurs as interaction between the individual and his environment.

Levels of Organization. Earlier you were told that the organism is related to its environment, the physical world, in several distinctly different ways. Four different levels of description are possible in depicting these organism-environment relationships. The first level or sort of interrelationship is the physical, in which the organism functions as any other material object. It may be heated, cooled, compressed, torn asunder just as any other substance. We do not very often have occasion to deal with the organism at this level, but for classification purposes it is very necessary to recognize the existence of this level. It ought to be easy to see that the human being is a part of nature at this level.

The second level is the biochemical, in which chemical processes as such are dealt with. At this level, the interrelation between the organism and its surrounds is through materials taken into the body, and to which the body reacts as a complex chemical system.

The next level important to us is the level at which tissues and organs are studied as such. This is generally thought of as physiology proper, though all studies of body process are thought of in a broad sense as physiology.

The level just above the specific tissue and organ level, is the homeostatic level. At this level, the organism is studied in a different way. Here one is concerned with what happens to the organism and what the organism does in response to various influences imposed upon it, such as temperature changes in the environment or such as the intake of specific substances into the body. The task of the organism is to maintain a high degree of constancy in a number of respects, despite external influences to the contrary. Most of homeostasis is expressed in chemical terms, although descriptions include what organs and tissues do, even some of the sense organs, to be mentioned at the next level. Since more than single organ systems are the points of interest, the homeostatic level is considered "higher' than the organ and tissue level.

The fifth and highest level is the sensory-cognitive. Energies effecting the organism at this level have a very different significance than those at the lower levels just described. At this level we are concerned with the results of activating sense organs and the central nervous system into which they feed. It is through this complex of higher order processes that we see, hear, touch, taste and smell, etc., and are able to act as total integrated purposeful organisms. Via sense organ and brain, the human experiences a world made up of things. This is the experiential world, which although it is common to believe exists outside of the individual himself, has no existence for the individual unless he has functional sensory and central nervous systems. Since it is at this level that the individual reaches awareness and at which his thoughts, purposes and feelings are directly describable it is the level to which most common-sense (untechnical) verbalizations refer. Much of the description at the sensory-cognitive level, as it refers to the human, is in social terms. The organism at this level is a person.[1] Much of psychology tends to neglect

------

[1] A variety of words are used today to designate the human being. They are partial synonyms, but each bears a somewhat different set of connotations, and fits in where the others may not do so well. It is helpful if those connotations are specified here so that the reader will be in an optimal position for under-

the fact that organism is related to its surrounds at levels below the experiential, and thus fails to comprehend the processes that provide the basis for the experiential events.

Were one to provide a full description of the mechanism of fatigue, the task would be to follow through the activities at each level of organization as they appear as consequences at the next higher level. Or better still, begin with the phenomenon of local interest, such as fatigue and determine how the activities at the lower levels contribute to making it what it is. One would have to: (1) deal with the consequences of the physical factors, and then the biochemical; (2) indicate the sequence of metabolic processes, beginning with food and oxygen intake through the consequences of energy expenditure in various given tasks; (3) depict the results of these biochemical events as describable at the homeostatic level as broad adjustments within the organism that must occur to maintain constancies in the context of the body cells; (4) describe how various changes at

––––––

standing them in what follows. The terms are: person, individual, subject, observer, patient, organism.

Person is a term used when dealing with the various high level things we see people do, such as perceiving, thinking, planning, remembering, becoming, hoping, etc., etc. In common usage, the word, person has always involved shifting from dealing with a biological organism to an immaterial behaving unit which we say is mental and not really a part of the biological, or even the physical universe. Perhaps, few will admit holding this position, but it is perfectly certain that no other position has clearly come into common use. We have pointed out that the person is simply the total organism in action.

Individual is simply a term that is intended to be less emphatic in its descriptive implications, except that at times, it may be used to distinguish the single human from the group. Subject is the term used to indicate the individual when used in an experiment. Observer is used in the same manner, except that he is a subject who is not the "passive" person, but one who plays the role of a perceiver. Patient is an individual whose status is well understood. He is one who consults and/or is treated by a physician or who is a subject in a clinical investigation. Organism is a term that is generally used for a sub-human biological unit. But the word, of course, applies as well to the human. In fact it seems to be the most appropriate label for him when his body processes are being studied and/or discussed, and when his physical and biochemical relations to the world are being dealt with. To most people the word organism is strange and inappropriate. This need not be so for its connotations are the very ones that often need to be understood and brought into use, as in the present situation dealing with fatigue.

the biochemical and homeostatic levels result in the emergence of sensory discomfort through the medium of the interoception; (5) depict the results ensuing from the impingement of external energies on the exteroceptors. This latter is the study of the nervous system as it underlies, sensation, perception, thinking, learning, believing and expressing attitudes, etc. A good description of this step has not been achieved.

The task just described would be a huge one if fully carried out. The main purpose here is not to go into specific detail, but rather to point out the nature of the task of dealing with the mechanism of fatigue.

Body Process Underlies all Experiencing. At the sensory-cognitive level descriptions turn from direct statements about body processes to statements about feelings, sensations, attitudes, etc. Here it must be recognized that for every feeling, every sensory experience, every conscious attitude, there is a unique combination of body processes underlying it and accounting for it. So to talk about feelings etc., is not necessarily to deny underlying body-process and to begin to talk about something separate from body, called mind. These descriptions should be thought of as being on a par with speaking of muscle contractions, in terms of *reaching, walking, running,* etc. The only essential difference is that the body processes underlying running etc., are better understood than those that underlie the items we call sensations, thoughts, attitudes etc. The words sensation, attitude, etc., simply stand for the total body-process complexes at a given time and also refer to meaningful organism-environment relations.

This is to say that the words we use when we talk about "mental" phenomena (experiential phenomena) fulfill two functions. They imply biological processes and they imply relations between organisms and their surrounds.

Going on from this, we can say then that when we use the word fatigue, we are implying an identifiable experiential complex, a set of body processes underlying this complex, and an orientation toward demand of some sort.

Once the identifiable experiential complex called fatigue is adequately described, it is to be accounted for in the manner we have already indicated. This must be done in conjunction with the orientation of the individual to the task or activity at hand, else we are simply describing empty sensory experiences, etc., that are related to nothing. Body discomfort unrelated to activity and the organism's orientation to it is an abstraction that has no usefulness or relevance in the description of fatigue.

Organism-centered and Environment-centered Reference Points. Studying fatigue, involves the awareness and proper selection of what we shall call *reference points.* Two reference points are possible in dealing with the interaction of the organism with its surrounds. The more usual reference point is the environment. The environment can be described more easily than the organism and very often it can be quantified. Studying the behavior or organisms in this way consists in relating its reactions to a describable set of conditions in the environment. We speak of this as the use of an environment-centered scheme.

It is also possible to use the organism as the reference. Organism-centered schemes are fairly rare, but some thinkers have come to believe that their use is quite necessary in dealing with certain problems. Fatigue is one of these. This requirement stems from the fact that the organism at the sensory-cognitive level is able to structure many ways of reacting to fixed external conditions. Organisms can assume unpredicted relationships to the environment.

Demand. Another of the major concepts that is needed in dealing with fatigue is demand. Demand is definable from either of the two reference points just described. Demand from the environmental standpoint is the requirement described by someone other than the performer himself. Demand from the organism's standpoint is the requirement the performer makes of himself. Even when stated in the same set of words by both the performer and the outsider requiring the task, the actual response called for may not be the same.

In order to account for what the performer does (succeeds or fails), the organism must be used as the reference. It is only to the degree that we can arrive at a picture of how the world looks to the performer, that we can make rime and reason out of his behavior. Clinically, this has often been the approach, but it certainly has not been in experimental research.

Cost. Cost is another concept that is useful in studying response of the individual to demand. It is far more common to measure work output than it is to measure cost to the performer. But for those who wish to study the organism as a performer, cost is quite pertinent.

Cost is expressed in several ways. The most usually dealt with form of cost is direct cost in physical energy, as measured in foot-pounds of work, or in calories, for example. Cost accrues in other forms. One of these is disorganization in the performer. Performance is an active ongoing affair and it does not leave the performer unaltered as activity continues. Change in functional interrelation between various component processes within the body occurs as activity goes on. In the case of skill, it is obvious that these activity components must occur in proper amounts and in the proper temporal relation to each other. Awkwardness and failure are the results when the proper working relations between parts fail to be maintained. This change we call *disorganization.* Disorganization is possible not only in skill, where complex neuromuscular activity is involved, but it is possible in the body processes underlying thinking, remembering, etc., and when it occurs it precludes the kind of accomplishment desired. Disorganization is involved in all forms of inadequacy. Disorganization is just as effective in reducing or precluding work output as is the lack of energy resources themselves. In accounting for some result the crucial feature is often not the lack of raw resources, but rather the nature of organization of processes which utilize energy.

Costs accrue at various levels of organization within the organism, and may thus be described in keeping with the language used for the particular level involved. Costs accruing at lower levels affect what accrues at higher levels of organization. In turn, costs accruing at the sensory-cognitive levels are reflected at lower levels. The manner in which the interactions occur is so complex and the temporal interrelations so extended that the delineation of what goes on is quite difficult.

Motivation. Motivation is another concept that is common in the study of behavior, and one that pertains to fatigue. Any behavior seems to involve two sets of relationships to the environment. One is given in the mere description of the immediate interactions themselves. The other is expressed in terms of goals, value systems, and other long-term contextual considerations. For example, some behavior may be inherent and immediately satisfying. It seems immediately gratifying for its own sake. Other forms of behavior will never occur unless there is some sort of a "reward" beyond the immediate outcome. This is well known, and those requiring certain kinds of performances from others seek to include strong rewards not inherent in the immediate situations. This whole process is called motivating the performer. The question of how to employ effective motivating factors looms large in getting many kinds of work done, particularly in prolonged tasks for it is in prolonged activity that body discomfort and other untoward body-process factors accumulate as activity continues. These weigh against whatever rewards there are.

The fact that we must reckon with is that much of the influence of the surrounds upon the individual operate at a verbal level, or at least at the social level, i.e., between the individual and other people in the many ways they have of interacting as persons. This means fatigue may be induced, or alleviated by things that people say to each other. In the common sense sphere this is known. It remains for formal science to envisage this category of influence so as to make it a part of biology, and not simply an empty take-over from common sense.

The Concept of Stress. Over the past several decades, a remarkable picture of the organism in reaction to demand has been developed through the thinking and research of a now well known endocrinologist, Dr. Hans Selye (51). The picture is of a condition which he calls *stress*. Stress not only illustrates the functional relation between levels of organization within the organism, but more especially the effects of demand on the organism. What Selye describes as stress and what we describe as fatigue have something in common as far as pattern of inducement is concerned. In both stress and fatigue, we are dealing with the reaction of the organism to conditions that tend to disrupt the balanced routine of the body.

We shall first indicate what Selye has found and what he has interpreted from it before we relate stress to what we have been calling fatigue. Here again, we are faced with using certain old words with new meanings. Stress, in older terminology, means that which disrupts or puts some sort of load or tension on an active system. In the new meaning, stress is the name for the condition produced, not the agent producing it. The agent is called a stressor.

Selye found that an endless variety of things may disrupt body function or be injurious to tissue. The results do not stop at the site of the application of the stressor, i.e., at the target organ or tissue. Tissue that is affected seems to be able to send into the blood stream some sort of a signal which reaches the master gland, the pituitary, which in turn reacts to set into motion certain influences on the adrenals and other endocrine glands. The hormones from these set into operation certain general tissue effects, making the end result (adaption) quite general rather than only local and specific.

Selye arrived at his concept of stress by several steps. To begin with he puzzled over the fact that the early stages of all illnesses have many features in common. The symptoms in all individuals are so nearly alike at first that diagnosis cannot be made. In the early stages of quite diverse diseases, the chief and almost only significant thing that can be said is, that the patients *are sick*. Being sick consists both in the way the patient feels, and in the anomalous functions detected by the physician.

Investigation into body process showed Selye that a characteristic triad of body changes are manifested in stress. The triad consists in adrenal enlargement, thymico-lymphatic involution and intestinal disturbance. This triad was seen to be the end result of an extended series of physiological events by which the body as a tissue system prepares itself to cope with the untoward influences bearing upon it. The extreme picture just implied in the triad does not often fully develop, but the initial stages leading up to the end result may occur again and again in life. Stress is truly unavoidable. Curiously enough, the influences called stressors are not all unpleasant. Many times they are the things we actively seek, and find most gratifying. This, of course, depends upon the value systems of the individuals involved.

Stressors include exertional activity as in sports, excitement, happiness, unhappiness, etc. They include physical conditions such as cold, heat, wounds, etc.

The body as a tissue system has a characteristic way of reacting when the alarm signal is given. While the sequence of bodily events alluded to above may serve to combat tissue insult, it is not apparent that these reactions are always very appropriate for they are initiated not only by insults to tissue such as in temperature extremes, but also by impulses from the sensory-cognitive system which has just received signals from the external environment. Thus the human organism at this advanced stage of evolution is equaly effected by influences that impinge upon its sense organs and operate at the sensory-cognitive level and by those at the biochemical and those which are the physical. The reactive machinery that the human possesses is the bodily machinery developed in its earlier evolutionary stages when there was no true sensory-cognitive system.

If the organism could now ignore what it hears or sees it would go unaffected by many things that now disequilibrate it (produce stress). The sensory mechanisms are, however, devices which often enable adjustments to the environment before extreme physical conditions take their toll.

It is crucial for the individual to possess a sort of sophistication and a "philosophy" that precludes unwholesome usages (interpretations) of external events which are made known through the senses. To the degree that this is possible certain occasions of stress are not brought about.

Since the impulses from the cortex, unlike signals from other tissue, may actually have nothing to do with tissue injury, the endocrine processes needed for repair of tissue are an inappropriate consequence.[2] Nevertheless the two diverse signal

---

[2] As a sidelight on the possibilities of cerebral influence on the rest of the body, we can point out that it has been just recently pretty well demonstrated that the apparent output of the brain when stimulated by such input pathways

sources are inherent in the human organism and both evoke the same initial reaction, which in turn sets up the same chain of consequences. Without the evolutionary development you have just been reminded of it is not evident why humiliation and subjection to extreme cold should evoke the same chain of internal body processes.

Stress and Fatigue. We introduced the concept and phenomena of stress here as an example of the fact that an influence entering the organism via sensory channels and thus at the sensory-cognitive level can produce a chain of consequences describable as body processes—in fact, the same set of consequences as when local tissue is insulted in some way. This is the same principle that applies in the case of fatigue. Selye's description of stressors and stress (including sensory-cognitive origins of stress) is a paramount example of science's progress beyond the common sense dualistic description of the human being and his environment.

As far as actual descriptions are concerned it could be expected that stress and fatigue have considerable in common. Stress, as Selye describes it, is depicted at the biochemical and physiological level. Fatigue as we describe it is depicted at the sensory-cognitive level. When fatigue is induced by certain frustrating circumstances, or prolonged unpleasant activity, evidently what Selye calls stress exists, too. To see the matter from the opposite side, when stress occurs, fatigue as a self-evaluative complex is likely to emerge, the necessary condition being the individual's self-recognition that he is not achieving as expected, or that his discomfort is attributable to his activity.

Being a biochemist, Selye is focally concerned with body processes at the biochemical level, leaving only logical room for descriptions at the sensory-cognitive level by those who see fit to make them explicit without escaping the biological and

------

as the vagus nerve may be not only neural but chemical. Stomach contractions have been produced in experimental preparations in which the only connection to the brain was the vagus, and the only avenue or influence from the brain was circulatory. We mention this here so as not to overlook the possible second avenue of the brain's influence on the rest of the body.

energistic world. Conventional descriptions have not met these requirements. Instead, they have developed from common sense and theistic origins, imputing (treating as fact) the existence of a non-material, non-biological entity called mind as the author of awareness in all its forms.

We are attempting to follow through on an outlook which provides a unitary natural account of all events, regardless of the level of description involved.

CHAPTER FIVE

The Chemistry of Fatigue

As the book title indicates, one of our major purposes is to deal with chemistry as related to fatigue. This chemistry refers first to certain descriptions of body process, and second to the question of what chemical substances, if any, may be used to prevent or alleviate fatigue.

That there are alterations in body process that lead to the individual's self-realization of inability to continue activity, there is no doubt. That the inability to carry on is in large part determined by the individual's cognitive assessment of himself including the discomfort involved is also clear.

As will be seen in the next chapter, there is a difference of opinion in regard to whether there are any pharmaceutical preparations on hand today suitable for the treatment of fatigue. This difference of opinion, no doubt, arises from wide differences in opinion as to what fatigue is and from differences in outlook on biology in general.

Ways of Altering Body Chemistry. The chemistry of the body may become altered by several means: (1) by body activity itself; (2) by changes in the environment such as temperature or humidity extremes; (3) by substances that are ingested or injected; or by deprivation of substances needed by the organism, such as oxygen, sugar, water, etc.

Activity alters the system that acts. These alterations are of two sorts, improvement toward a criterion, which is *learning*, and impoverishment, which has often been called *fatigue*, but which is more appropriately called *impairment*.

Fatigue, as we define it, may or may not result from impairment. In some cases, no fatigue occurs because the impairment so involves the central nervous system that the individual is temporarily made unable to adequately evaluate his own acts and his relation to the environment. Oxygen deprivation, sedation, and alcoholic and other forms of intoxication are examples. In other cases, the individual is not at the moment doing anything in particular and is unaware of what he would not be able to do if he tried.

There are many situations that do impair certain forms of body process, such as muscle activity, or that produce body discomfort. When discomfort arises in the midst of a task, fatigue is likely to ensue.

The Chemistry of Fatigue. The chemistry that we shall call the chemistry of fatigue refers to several things: (1) the chemistry of metabolism, primarily that of foods, in which the ability to metabolize at sufficient rates during exertion is crucial; (2) the chemistry that has to do with mood; (3) the chemistry of the hormonal system which is a part of the chemistry involved in the maintenance of health; (4) the chemistry involved in activation of interoceptors which relay tissue condition to the sensory-cognitive centers of the brain.

It is not to be taken for granted by the reader that all the chemistry implied above is yet known, and even if it were, that we would have space or reason to go into detail about it. What will be said will be brief and superficial.

Carbohydrate Metabolism. Carbohydrate metabolism includes all of the reactions in the body undergone by carbohydrates after ingestion and also by the carbohydrates formed in the body from other sources. These include starch and glycogen, the polysaccharides; maltose, sucrose, and lactose, the disaccharides; and glucose, fructose, and galuctose, the monosaccharides; and certain other substances. The disaccharides and the polysaccharides, with the exception of lactose and glycogen are hydrolyzed to monosaccharides in the alimentary canal. Accordingly the processes of intermediate metabolism primarily involve the monosaccharides. The compounds formed are glycogen, pyruvic acid, lactic acid, and acetic acid. These are three of the commonest substances intermediate between glucose and carbon dioxide and water as end products. Many other intermediate substances are involved as well.

Blood sugar (blood glucose) is the form in which carbohydrate is taken to various parts of the body by the circulation. As the blood flows through the gut, the blood glucose concentration is raised; as it flows through other tissues blood glucose is withdrawn. The level is kept relatively constant by the liver which is able to turn glucose into glycogen when in excess in the blood, or to convert glycogen and some of the amino acids back into blood glucose when the blood concentration is low.

In muscle cells, glucose provides the chemical energy for contraction. Skeletal muscle is able to synthesize glycogen from glucose and to store it as a carbohydrate reserve. From 0.5 to 1.0 per cent of muscle weight may consist in this energy reserve.

The breakdown of glycogen in muscle for use is somewhat like the process in the liver, and a series of reactions occur which finally yields pyruvic and lactic acid. There are two paths of utilization, the aerobic and anaerobic. The anaerobic yields lactic acid with an energy content of nine-tenths of the original glucose. Lactic acid, unless it can be used, will deprive the body of considerable energy whenever muscle functions under anaerobic conditions. There seem to be two ways this lactic may be used. In the presence of oxygen, it may be oxidized back to pyruvic acid in muscle, or it may be resynthesized to glycogen. Since lactate is highly diffusible it may pass into the blood or lymph and reach the liver which may resynthesize it into glycogen.

Most of the intermediate substances of muscle metabolism are present in muscle most any time but have limited diffusibility. Little appears in the blood stream. Lactic and pyruvic acids, however, are quite diffusible, especially when muscle is functioning under anaerobic conditions. Anaerobic conditions eventuate during strenuous muscle activity, or even when less activity is involved, if the individual's oxygen supply is reduced, such as at high altitudes.

Lactic acid begins to accumulate in the blood whenever oxygen supply is insufficient. There is a limit to the total amount tolerated and this is in the neighborhood of 130 grams. In some forms of muscular activity the rate of accumulation may reach 3 grams per second. Obviously this limits the duration of such activity, as for example, the time during which no breathing may occur. A concentration of thirty times normal has been reported, under strenuous exercise. After termination of a bout of exercise with inadequate oxygen supply, lactic acid continues to escape into the blood for awhile. The anaerobic level remains for possibly eight minutes, and complete return to normal may require one-half to one and one-half hours. The liver is the chief organ involved in the restoration. In extremely strenuous exercise, the kidneys eliminate a small amount of the blood lactic acid.

Lipid Metabolism. Fat is taken into the blood stream directly and remains in circulation for sometime, from which it is withdrawn by the tissues which are involved in lipid metabolism. Fats, of course, contain more energy, per unit weight than either proteins or carbohydrates. When food intake is excessive, the excess products are stored as fat mainly in adipose tissue. While the organism lives entirely on stored proteins and fats during fasting periods, it likewise uses some lipids during the usual every day course of events.

Lipids are transported by the plasma of the blood. The blood fatty acid content is made up of three kinds of substances, neutral fat, cholesteral esters, and phospholipid and glycerol. The total cholesterol content is part free, and part esterified.

Lipids absorbed from the alimentary canal are involved in three consequencies, one of which is storage in adipose tissue. Later they may be used in the body for heat and energy. For this, two pathways seem to be open. The first is direct utilization.

The second path for lipid use begins in a way similar to the first. In its course ketone bodies are formed. They are readily formed in the liver but are utilized there only slightly. When this concentration rises high they defuse into the hepatic sinusoids producing ketonemia. Ketonemia becomes greater at times when the body is deriving most of its energy and heat from lipid breakdown as in starvation, or in diabetes mellitus. One of the difficulties produced by the keto acids is the disturbance of the mechanisms that regulate acid-base balance in the body, bringing about acidosis.

Protein Metabolism. Protein use involves two phases. The first stage occurs in the alimentary canal. Here certain enzymes in the digestive juices break the complex proteins molecules into amino acids or to the peptides, simple chains of animo acids. These are absorbed by the blood and lymph. The liver and peripheral tissues remove and store considerable amounts of them.

The gut is not the only source of amino acids entering the portal blood stream. They are constantly being interchanged between the blood and the kidney, liver, spleen and skeletal muscle. During fasting or starvation, the preponderance is in the direction of yielding amino acids to the blood stream.

Most of the amino acid supply is made into protein, oxidized to carbon dioxide, urea and water, changed to carbohydrate or fat, or utilized to form certain derivatives, for example, creatine, epinephrine, glutathione, etc.

While protein as well as carbohydrate and fat can be utilized for muscular energy, only about 2 per cent of the energy is generally obtained from protein.

Shifts in the proportions of carbohydrate and fats being used occur during different rates and prolongations of work. In light activity the proportions of fat and carbohydrates is about the same as with the individual at rest, namely about two-thirds from fat and one-third from carbohydrate (not counting the slight protein contribution). As the rate of energy utilization increases, the proportion of energy derived from carbohydrate rises. On the other hand, if strenuous exercise is prolonged, the reserve carbohydrate supply (in liver and muscle) may become short or exhausted, and force the muscles to obtain their energy from fat. When this trend runs to extremes, exhaustion and collapse may occur (as in marathon races) probably because of functional impairment of the central nervous system which requires a certain supply of carbohydrate (glucose) at all times.

Fluid Balance in Exercise. The water content of the average person is about 70 per cent. The actual percentage varies inversely with the individual's fat content since fat is not accompanied by a corresponding amount of water. Water is contained in intra cellular and extra cellular compartments. Extra cellular compartments are of two sorts, vascular and interstitial.

Exchange of fluids between blood and interstitial spaces occurs in the capillaries of the circulatory system. Under normal resting conditions filtration and reabsorption of fluid at the arterial and venous ends of capillaries balance. When so, tissue fluid volume is constant. Exercise is one of the factors which disturbs this balance. When filtration of fluids out of the capillaries is greater than its reabsorption, edema results. If the balance is disturbed in the opposite direction dehydration ensues. Shift in salt balance may change the amount of fluids within the cells.

Shifts in posture from reclining to erect position alter fluid balance, producing "dependent edema" after excessive periods of standing. Single strenuous bouts of exercise causes excess fluid to leave the blood. This causes what is called hemoconcentration. Sweating during the bout will add to the hemoconcentration.

Chronic exercise in the trained subject seems not to produce sustained shifts in fluid balance. Bouts of strenuous exercise may cause dehydration and this, of course, has unfavorable results, such as loss in blood volume, rise in rectal temperature and pulse rate and earlier onset of exhaustion.

Other Aspects of Metabolism. In addition to the foregoing features of metabolism, there are other forms involving the utilization of vitamins, minerals etc.

The production of enyzmes is one important aspect of body economy. The enzymes are biological chemical catalysts and if they were always present when and where needed many functional difficulties in the body's chemical machinery would not exist. Apparently some individuals do not manufacture certain useful enzymes, and their absence makes for certain distressing difficulties There is some evidence to indicate that the absence of some enzymes is genetically determined. The fact that individuals do differ in their enzymetic resources helps to account for many symptoms that people have long complained of but which could not be well accounted for and were attributed to "imagination." In cases in which certain enzymes are lacking, the resources of the individuals are limited either directly or through secondary avenues of discomfort etc.

Training in Physical Fitness. While descriptions of the metabolism of various foods, minerals, vitamins, etc. indicate the major features of metabolism, they may not fully disclose the relative importance of the various components involved in the metabolic chain. One of the ways to discover this is to determine what goes on in the individual that can best perform strenuous tasks, or considerable work over long periods as in contrast to the metabolic pattern of those who cannot. The crucial differences between the unfit and the fit are made manifest through training processes. Training or the development of fitness is brought about by simply requiring progressively greater amounts of exertion. During the course of this training some metabolic processes change little, others considerably more. The importance of the processes that change as a consequence of training is thereby inferable. The investigator is given a picture of the differences between adequate and inadequate patterns of metabolism for exertion. Much of the information about changes produced by training in physical fitness consists in descriptions of the differences in the ways the lungs, heart, circulation and other organs and systems function before and after. This sort of information will be omitted here since it is not given in chemical terms.

Chemical Changes Produced by Exercise and Training. The following are some of the changes in physical fitness brought about by training. Strenuous training appears to increase total blood hemoglobin and blood volume. Not all types of training seemed to do this and from the facts at hand it has been concluded that frequent bouts of very vigorous exercise involving hypoxic conditions are necessary. While total hemoglobin may increase, relative hemoglobin tends to remain constant with exercise.

The count of red blood cells is often increased in the early stages of exertion. This may be due to hemoconcentration, i.e., the transfer of fluid from the circulatory system to the tissues. After longer exercise, net fluid exchange reverses, providing a dilution which would naturally lower the cell count per unit volume. Extreme exertion may increase the rate of red cell destruction from capillary compression by muscles and from increased velocity of blood flow. These effects would be more likely in sporadic bouts in sedentary individuals than in the more completely trained individual.

There is also some evidence that while extra-cellular fluids remain constant, intra-cellular water and total body water increases with the training. Apparently levels of blood lactate following sub-maximal exercise, tend to be inversely reportional to the degree of fitness of the individual. The ability of the individual to tolerate higher concentrations of blood lactate before exhaustion increases with fitness.

There is evidence that training reduces the amount of oxygen required by working muscles. If, as a consequence, blood flow to the muscles is reduced, there is more blood available for other tissues, assuming the same cardiac output. But the ability to consume more oxygen during strenuous exercise is increased and there is a greater ability to utilize anaerobic energy reserves.

It has been shown that at high work levels, for a given minute volume of air, oxygen intake and carbon dioxide output increase with training. For a given ventilation more oxygen is taken up by the trained individual than by the untrained.

Blood cholesterol levels can be reduced by exercise while keeping diet constant. This lasts only while training is continued. The cholesterol reduction is thought to be due to increased fat mobilization and utilization during exercise.

Albuminuria as a result of strenuous exercise disappears with training. This may be a result of more blood being available to the kidneys as training progresses.

Digestion and Exertion. It has generally been believed that exertion interfers with digestion, but this has been studied by investigating the influence of exertion on gastric secretion and stomach peristalisis. Brief vigorous, and extended taxing exertion inhibit the secretion of acid, and gastric peristalisis both during and for a short time following exertion. It seems as though a period of hyperactivity then sets in. Mild exertion seems not to effect secretion and motility very greatly. Training seems to diminish the vigor of the stomach reactions just described.

Intestinal motility has not been similarly investigated but it would seem likely that exertion does effect it. While it has been concluded that exertion, in most cases has little negative effect on digestion, trainers seem to have evidence to the contrary. Interference with the diaphragm by stomach distention tends to lead to the diminished efficiency of the respiratory system.

As yet, the effect of exertion on the chemistry of digestion has not been fully determined by experimental methods, but no doubt, in sedentary and older individuals, the factors of exertion and routine tension do certainly upset digestion, which is to say changes its overall chemistry in certain ways.

Fatigue. The metabolic (chemical) basis for fatigue results from the undue demands upon the processes of metabolism. What constitutes an undue demand is more likely to be some sudden increase in exertion for which the individual is not trained than merely strenuous activity itself. Significant fatigue stemming from metabolic factors is more likely to appear in the individual of purely sedentary habits than among those given to moderate routine exertion. As age increases, however, the ability to reach a fair amount of fitness following a long period of sedentary living seems to decrease. At least the improvement becomes slower and not so likely to be as great.

Chemistry of the Hormone System. One aspect of the activity of the hormone system was discussed in the preceding chapter in dealing with Selye's description of stress. This, to some extent, obviates the necessity of so much being said at this point.

The chief thing to concern us here is what Selye (51) says

about the way the body meets the great variety of insults against it, for example, anything from exposures to atom bombs, the effects of over-exertion, to insect bites. He points out that the way the body meets these is by the production of *inflammation.* Virtually any agent can induce inflammation in most any part of the body, and with quite varied results. "Inflammation," he points out, "is a reaction to injury." In being this, it is an active result, not a mere passive affair. The Romans provided, what has ever since been the essential description of inflammation—redness and swelling, heat and pain. Of course, interference of function is a fifth characteristic. Inflammation is not only a defense reaction but is involved in tissue repair. But like other forms of defense in systems even outside the body, it may sometimes impose self-inflicted injury as it plays its role.

The hormones are the regulators of this defense, some being pro-inflammatory, and others anti-inflammatory in their function. ACTH which is discharged by the pituitary induces the adrenals to make anti-inflammatory substances (A-Cs), such as cortisone and cortisol. Something else induces the adrenals to form pro-inflammatory substances (P-Cs). The amounts of A-Cs and P-Cs in the blood can vary independently. To change the consequences of given balances between the two, it is not always necessary to change the existing proportions between them. If considerable of the two are in the blood, the A-Cs are always the more effective. In other words, with the existence of considerable A-C, no amount of P-C is effective in balancing it out.

Another way of changing the degree of inflammability is through the production of a pituitary secretion that inhibits the effects of ACTH. Such a substance is STH, the growth hormone, also called the somatotropic hormone. It is not too clear how STH acts and it is not necessary here that we know. Our purpose is only to remind the reader that hormones have to do with the maintenance of normal tissue functions, i.e., body health, and that exertion can be one of the stressors to set up inflammation when the individual's exertion exceeds the amount the muscular system has been adapted (trained) to. Over-exertion can be a stressor and produce the same effects that other stressors do.

One of the many things to remember here is that the mechanism involved in the defense of a specific set of tissues may set up consequences that go beyond the specific tissues directly involved. Something consequently happens in a variety of tissues throughout the body. It is in this way that what happens to the organisms is seldom, if ever, exclusively local. Sometimes the pervasive effect is not intense enough to cause overall results that are significant in modifying performance on the personalistic level but often it is. One of the effects is the production of body discomfort or reduced effectiveness in performance. Thus fatigue as we have defined it, is one of the consequences.

Not all hormone activity is directly related to inflammation. During exercise, supposedly there is, for example, an increase in the secretion of the antidiuretic hormone (ADH). Consequently there is a greater reabsorption of fluid from the renal tubules and thus a reduction in urine formation.

Heavy exertion, anxiety etc., increase the secretion of the adrenal cortex resulting in a reduction of the eosinophils in the blood. The peak of the effect occurs usually several hours after the application of the stressor. Associated with the effect on eosinophils, is a decrease in the number of lymphocytes and an increase in neutrophils.

Chemistry as Related to Mood. Mood is related to the discussion of fatigue in several ways. Individuals in depression are not generally able to perform well. They do not want to work, nor do they accomplish much when they attempt to meet the demands upon them. On the other side of the picture, there are times in which mood is elevated rather than depressed. In such cases, desire for activity and accomplishment is high, exertion does not seem to take toll, and a favorable view is taken of everything, including accomplishment that at other times would not be judged too promising. In this latter state performance may be maintained for longer periods, and the state called fatigue does not so readily supervene

All too little is known about the chemistry underlying mood, and not very much can be said. Mood, of course, is not something that is usually described in body-process terms. The vocabulary describing it has to do with matters of feeling, attitude, strength of motivation, etc. Nevertheless, body process underlies all moods, and it is body process that accounts for them.

The body processes most crucial to mood as is the case with all aspects of overall-behavior, are the processes that go on in the nervous system. In dealing with these, two main considerations are to be kept in mind. One is the fact that the central nervous system is endless in the patterns of activity possible even when no impairment is involved. The processes that constitute human cognition, attitudes etc., are accountable for partly in terms of this endless potentiality for variation Some activity of the central nervous system, on the other hand, is determined by certain deviations in body chemistry. This is to say that euphoria-depression; alertness-stupidity, sanity-insanity, urge-to-work-fatigue, etc., are partly expressions of the individual as arrived at through training, and partly, results of fortunate or unfortunate patterns of chemistry. The more difficult of the two factors to delineate in concerte terms is the potentiality for variety of action that is inherent in the system; the more concrete is the class of phenomena that can be dealt with through analysis of chemical deviations. An adequate grasp of either is far from having been achieved yet.

Most of the investigations of mood have not dealt with work aversion and fatigue, but other matters such as psychopathology, so there is all too little to report here. We can be sure, however, that there is a connection between brain chemistry, mood, and consequent fatigue.

Perhaps not all of mood stems directly from chemical conditions originating within the nervous system but rather from chemical factors that cause sensory inputs to be relayed to it from widespread tissues which are in certain degrees of difficulty.

Here we have reference to the conditions in tissue which involve chemical mediators, either by way of setting up afferent nerve impulses in widely scattered sense cells throughout the body, or transmitting substances which affect central nervous centers more or less directly.

Muscle Metabolism and Bodily Discomfort. There are two

possible channels through which the condition of muscles if relayed to the central nervous system so as to have an effect upon how the individual feels. The one channel would be the kinesthetic pathway over which we now know that information regarding various tension states of muscle is relayed to result in sensory effects. The other would involve the circulatory system. If the latter were involved, then substances put into the blood from muscle as it is exercised would find their way to some chemo-receptor upstream or would in some mysterious way affect certain brain centers directly. This, of course, is not in line with prevailing thought. However, Selye has demonstrated to his satisfaction that all tissues when insulted produce some chemical that the blood carries to the pituitary gland and starts a chain of consequences which he calls the General Adaptation Syndrome. More recently it has been shown that stimulation of the vagus afferents to the brain in an animal in which the vagus supply to the stomach is severed, produces gastric contractions, the avenue for inducing seeming to be the circulatory system (see footnote 2 in Chapter 4). This would mean that the brain causes some substance to be carried in the circulation.

Regardless of whether the state of muscles is made known through a neural or a chemical channel, it is certainly made known. It is entirely plausible that the metabolic state of muscle in being a chemical state is also expressed in mechanical terms. That is, that the chemical state effects the mechanical properties of muscle, and that the kinesthetic receptors in being mechanical receptors are able to discriminate certain mechanical differences in muscle in addition to the ones that have to do with the ordinary forms of muscle contraction. These mechanical activities may be unsteady or step-wise contractile patterns when muscles are in subnormal states, as in contrast to finely graded contraction patterns under normal circumstances. This difference in muscle activity if it existed could be the basis for sending differently distributed nerve impulse groupings to the brain, where they would be the basis for the individual's feeling firm, strong, steady and comfortable, or on the other hand weak, shaky, unsteady, and uncomfortable.

Some kind of further understanding of the results of muscle

metabolism as it pertains to the production of various forms of bodily discomfort is necessary in order to relate metabolism to feeling states of the individual. We are here only indicating in a speculative way but in a plausible way what the relation might be. This fulfills an obligation to the reader to suggest an avenue from body chemistry to body discomfort and thus the individual's self assessment of declining ability to carry on. Some experimental information about such an avenue must be obtained for no matter how much is said about body chemistry, two *results* of the chemistry of exertion have to be delineated: (1) the nature of the muscle's declining abilities, and (2) the relating of this decline to body feeling and its cognitive or personalistic end result, fatigue.

CHAPTER SIX

Agents Relieving Fatigue and Related Conditions

IN THIS CHAPTER, THE MORE PROMINENT AGENTS FOR RELIEVING STATES ASSOCIATED WITH FATIGUE, AND thus often fatigue itself, will be discussed. There is considerable difference of opinion regarding the efficacy of medicines for this purpose. The issue often centers on whether what helps relieve a condition associated with or underlying fatigue is to be considered as one relieving fatigue. Our position here is, that since one cannot easily disassociate the various components of an overall condition, whatever is known to help the general condition is close enough to relieving the symptom itself to be considered. Fatigue, although it can be identified, can scarcely be isolated from the conditions associated with it, and which often form a basis for it. Hence the preparations to be discussed in this chapter, although not offered as direct remedies for fatigue may well be thought relevant in the attempt to lessen or abolish it. The substances may apply, depending upon the nature of the overall condition of the individual. There is none of the medicines in the groups to be discussed but which has helped or failed to help depending upon the particular nature of the case.

To relieve fatigue, several things may be done: (1) one may relieve body discomfort; (2) enable muscular activity; (3) elevate mood; (4) improve metabolism in general; (5) counteract aging, and (6) improve outlook on life. All these measures are, of course, aside from providing rest and change. The question that we shall occupy ourselves with is whether pharmaceutical agents can help in accomplishing one or more of the results just listed.

The substances to be mentioned except in a very few instances, are those suggested in response to inquiries sent to a group of pharmaceutical companies asking whether they produced any preparations which might be useful in combating fatigue and associated symptoms. The answers were somewhat varied. Out of the thirty-three companies responding, twelve or more than 36 per cent, said they manufactured nothing of the sort, and several of them said that there is no known substance useful in treating fatigue. The remainder supplied information regarding preparations which may produce effects at least indirectly useful for this purpose.

Relief of Body Discomfort. One of the deterants to activity and continued performance is bodily discomfort. It is a salient basis for fatigue. Many required tasks produce it. Various sorts of activity while helping to maintain health and effectiveness, produce body discomfort in the form of muscular stiffness, aches and pains. Fatigue is generally the outcome when performance is maintained in the face of these. The question then is whether any substance can be taken to relieve this discomfort. If so, the lessening or preclusion of fatigue might be expected.

One of the most widely used substances presumably for relieving pain is aspirin. Many seemingly contradictory statements have been made regarding its worth. This is probably largely because there are various sorts of pain and therefore unrealistic expectations regarding its effectiveness. Possibly in spite of its very prevalent use, few people can say just what aspirin does for them. As a result it is easy to pass off aspirin as simply a substance that too many people have gotten into the habit of taking, regardless of results or regardless of need. Consequently any advocacy of aspirin here might seem to be inappropriate. This is not quite the case, however.

Aspirin is in the class of substances known as analgesics, and thus is supposed to relieve pain. There are two tests for any pain reliever, the report of the victim in everyday life, and the findings of controlled laboratory experiments. Apparently the effectiveness of aspirin and other substances to relieve pain is not actually accomplished in the manner supposed. In laboratory experiments, very often pain thresholds are studied. In such cases, it would be expected that analgesics would do their work by raising the threshold for pain. When so, the subject would require a stronger application of the pain producer than before in order to just feel minimal pain. It has been found that even morphine, one of the more powerful drugs in this respect, does not greatly affect the pain threshold. Apparently the effect is of a more general nature and has to do with more pervasive changes in the individual which alter the overall reaction to noxious stimuli rather than simply lessening the ability to feel the more direct result of disturbing local tissue. This principle applies to aspirin, and the relief that it provides (when it provides any) is to make the individual feel better in general. It is more nearly a comfort-producing agent than an effective pain-killer. In human subjects, aspirin seems to be about 1/30 as effective as morphine in relieving pain under certain of the conditions studied.

The idea that aspirin acts by antagonizing natural pain substances in the blood and other tissues of the body has led to a series of investigations. A certain class of peptides called kinins has been studied in this connection. Bradykinin supposedly excites nerve endings in the viscera leading to the experience of pain. In canine experiments it has been shown that aspirin blocks the action of bradykinin. Bradykinin produces overt responses in mice when injected into the abdominal cavity. Aspirin blocks this reaction.

It has also been shown that not all painful effects of bradykinin can be blocked by aspirin. It is known that itching of the skin produced by bradykinin is not prevented by aspirin, but it is prevented by morphine.

Aspirin has another worthwhile effect which may have some remote relation to body conditions underlying fatigue. It has a slight effect in counteracting anaphylactic shock. For example, kinins are one of two known substances involved in constricting the bronchioles of the guinea pig, and are involved in anaphylactic shock. Constriction of the bronchioles does not result, if a small dose of aspirin is given a few minutes beforehand. Apparently aspirin has no effect upon histamine, the more commonly recognized substance in untoward tissue reactions, although it does antagonize kinin and SRS-A, another substance involved in such reactions.

In general, it seems that aspirin plays a role in modifying the defense reactions to various kinds of stressors of body tissue, and in this respect is not to be too lightly thought of. It is probably in this way that it produces whatever bodily comfort it does.

To the extent that it improves general body comfort, it should be a help in lessening fatigue. It must be recognized that, in the case of aspirin as in the case of many other substances, the effect of prolonged usage is not fully known. Too many substances which seem to be effective during early usage become less effective as usage continues.

Improvement of Muscular Activity. Caffeine is another substance so common as to be almost needless to mention. Individuals react in various ways and degrees to it and anything that is said about its use would have to be directed in two ways. Suggestions would have to be different to pertain to daily coffee, tea, and cola users than to pertain to abstainers. In fact, many persons are already dependent upon caffeine, and in being so, possibly lose the benefit that may be obtained by abstainers who use it for medicine on special occasions.

What is known in regard to the possible differences in conditions of users and non-users is virtually negligible despite the widespread familiarity with caffeine beverages. Hence what we shall present here are only a few of the general facts usually given for caffeine.

Caffeine is said to increase "ease of muscular contraction." It increases the total energy output of muscle in experiments where muscle is stimulated directly. It increases the oxygen consumption of resting muscle many fold. Oxygen consumption in nerve is increased with weak concentrations and reduced in strong concentrations in laboratory experiments.

Certain early workers reported that caffeine increases the *amplitude* of muscle contraction in ergographic experiments but not the *number* of contractions needed to produce exhaustion. This led to the inference that caffeine primarily effected muscle rather than nervous tissue, since it was thought that the number of contractions reflected the state of the nervous system.

A variety of other studies ranging from those on both smooth and striated excised muscle to ergographic and dynameter studies on the intact subject have also led to the conclusion that caffeine has an activating effect on muscle tissue. Actually caffeine has additional effects among which are raising the excitability of the central nervous system, and producing vasodilation.

Caffeine can undoubtedly be classed as a substance relieving fatigue and improving work performance (26).

Elevation of Mood. Nothing describable as mood is generally involved in transient fatigue. But in chronic fatigue, tiredness is often associated with mood in the form of depression. Actually the physician may be as much or more concerned with mood as with tiredness. However, relief from tiredness or fatigue may be gained from doing something calculated to elevate mood. Even the term depression, though quite inclusive, is not always the whole picture. Agitation is often part of the syndrome. Since the syndrome is complex, different treatments center on different aspects or components. In our case, we are primarily interested in fatigue as one of them. Fatigue may not be easily isolated from the others.

Various drugs are available for elevating mood, but all of them are not equally effective. This makes for success and failures from physician to physician, and results which sometimes seem contradictory.

One of the chief groups of substances used for elevation of mood are the amphetamines. The amphetamines have come to be one of the classes of drugs quite widely used illegitimately and foolishly these days. They produce addiction with all its hazards and miseries. Benzedrine (amphetamine sulphate) was one of the earlier drugs to appear in recent years and was the object of experimental comparison with such substances as caffeine. It was from such studies that it was concluded that one positive effect of amphetamine was the shift in mood. This drug is said by some to be variable in its effects from person to person. Paradoxical effects such as forgetfulness, dullness, increase in fatigue, malaise and drowsiness have been reported. It increases motor activity in some cases and decreases it in others. Some report that the drug increases confidence, initiative, and ease in making decisions, and even produces euphoria.

Table I lists the more prominent amphetamines which are used today, either alone or in compounds. The table is restricted by the fact that the list contains only the examples suggested by their makers for use in connection with fatigue and depression. Not all pharmaceutical companies would class these compounds as useful for fatigue and related difficulties.

The amphetamines are considered stimulants. In fact, drugs whose net result is excitation are called either psychic energizers, stimulants, or anti-depressants.

Himwich (25) points out that although psychiatric usage treats the words stimulant, energizer and anti-depressant as synonyms, such drugs may be put into two categories. Those of the one class *increase* the electrical activity of the brain and may be called psychic energizers. Many of them are analeptics. In this group are the amphetamines, ephedrine, methylphenidate, piprodrol, iproniazid, and dimethylaminoethanol. These have to do with the alerting reaction, a response said to require more energy than spontaneous activity.

In the second category are methylphenidate and benactyzine, which *inhibit* the reticular formation, thereby supposedly reducing the effect of what would otherwise be disagreeable stimulation. This holds for reduction in disturbing beliefs as well as sensory material.

Another substance, d-desoxyephedrine, also known as Pervitin is somewhat like Benzedrine in its effects, with possibly a greater toxicity, and with smaller amounts required to obtain similar effects.

A number of anti-depressant substances or components excluding the amphetamines are listed in Table II. These are now used by some physicians in place of amphetamines. Accordingly we shall indicate what some writers have to say about them.

Ritalin (methlphenidate hydrochloride) is an anti-depressant which is said to improve mood and performance, and is suggested by some in treating fatigue and mild depression states, and lethargy due to illness etc. However, when anxiety is present, it may intensify it. Given orally, it seldom produces blood pressure changes. Like many other substances used to stimulate or depress, it produces side effects or may not prove the right drug for certain patients. Ritalin has been used by many physicians and a number of them have written about it.

Elavil is a compound of amitriptyline chloride, dextrose, methylparaben, and propylparaben in aqueous solution, which is given parentrally. It is said to have a low degree of toxicity. It is not an amine oxidase inhibitor as are some of the other substances in this class. It has both anti-depressant and tranquilizing properties. In some cases Elavil has been used in preference to electric shock therapy.

It would seem that while Elavil is classed as a psychic energizer, the chief effect is that of sedation and allaying agitation, a predominant and troublesome component or associate of some forms of depression.

Amitriptyline was studied as a comparison substance to the amphetamines, and meprobamate by Holliday and Devery who concluded that whereas amitriptyline may be an effective anti-depressant, it is not in itself an effective "anti-fatigue" agent. Fatigue in this case was synonymous to performance decrement, not the experienced inadequacy we mean.

Deaner (deanol) the para-acetamidobenzoic acid salt of (2-dimethylaminoethanol) is one of the newer psychic energizers. A number of physicians, including Lemere (31, 32), Settel (52), Snow (55), Tracy (58), and Young (63), have published in its favor. Deanol is neither a monoamine oxidase inhibitor nor a sympathomimetic substance.

Lemere (32) states that certain anti-depressant properties

claimed for several of the tranquilizers, for instance, mepazine (Pactal), meprobamate plus benactyzine (Deprol) have not in his opinion been proven. He suggests Deaner as a psychic energizer. This substance is a promoter of the formation of acetylcholine in the brain and the facilitation of nervous activity. He points out that after a year's use, it has proved better for his depressed patients than the amphetamines. It seems to be without side effects except the feelings of overstimulation when the dosage is high. However, it has been of no use in the treatment of severe depressions. Since our interest here is in dealing with persons who are mildly depressed and whose symptoms include fatigue as a symptom, it would seem to be a possibility.

Meller (37) distinguishes between two forms of depression, the severe, which is often dealt with by more heroic methods such as electric shock therapy and the mild which is associated with fatigue and frequent headaches. There seems to be two different neurophysiologic mechanisms involved. The patients with mild depression respond to Deaner.

Moriarty and Mebane (38, 39) point out that although the clinical effects of Deaner are not marked with modest doses, they are impressed by the type of stimulation produced when given in sufficient amounts. It produces a natural effect in contrast to the apparently artificial type produced by amphetamine. Along with this there seems to be no dangerous or unpredictable complications as seen with certain other substances such as iproniazid. These authors also discriminate between patients who are the common candidates for electric shock treatment and the milder type which Deaner benefits. The effects are roughly comparable to those of hormones or vitamin-like substances which exist naturally in the body but which may be in deficient supply. They say that Deaner is especially useful in chronic fatigue states.

Settel (52) finds Deaner useful for patients of all ages for mild depression, reserving iproniazid for the severely depressed institutionalized individual. Snow *et al.* (55) recommend Deaner for chronic fatigue states, mild depressions, and neurasthenia. Tracy (58) obtained fair to excellent results on a group of his patients suffering what he calls a cyclic psychosomatic fatigue syndrome. In some of his cases in which many other substances such as Dexedrine, Ritalin, Methedrine etc. failed, Deaner's effects were encouraging.

Young (63) says that the mood elevating effects of Deaner are definite but gradual and subtle. As a result they may not be noticed unless attention is paid and treatment is continued for several weeks.

Stelazine (trifluoperazine) is a substance classed as a central nervous depressant. It has been mainly used in the treatment of psychoneurotic symptoms. Those who have reported on it included May, Whitely and Gradwell (35); Rowell and Segal (50); Gearren (20); Maerz, Lee and Hunter (34). The drug seems to be useful in patients with tension, and has been found useful in obsessional personalities, when chloropromazine has not proved successful. While this substance is not one for use in a direct attack on fatigue it may be beneficial in certain cases in which fatigue and tension are associated symptoms.

Deprol (benactyzine hydrochloride plus meprobamate) is a compound that has its advocates despite the fact that others who have used it have turned to something they find better for relief of the symptoms at hand. Deprol is advocated as being most effective in acute situational and reactive depressions of moderate degree. Those who have used it and have written about it include Alexander (1), Beerman (12), Gordon (21), McClure (36), and Rickels and Ewing (45).

Benactyzine, a component of Deprol, is sometimes manufactured as Suavitil. Benactyzine was first used treating patients with anxiety and depression. It is supposed to elevate what is sometimes called the emotional threshold. Tension springing from conflict between patient and surroundings was said to be relieved quite well. Two main side reactions reported have been general apathy or detachment and anomalous sensations in the limbs.

Pharmacologically benactyzine is a spasmolitic as tested on isolated intestine and is also a weak antihistamine. It has also a variety of other pharmacological effects as tested on laboratory preparations. It suppresses alpha waves in the EEG and is somewhat analgesic. Meprobamate, the other ingredient of Deprol, is a tranquilizer, a muscle relaxent and anticonvulsant.

Some physicians report low toxicity of Deprol, while others warn against the use of benactyzine and the tranquilizers.

Anabolic Agents. Various substances have a positive effect on certain metabolic processes and are called anabolic agents. The following are examples.

Adroyd (oxymetholone) is a substance useful in states of asthenia and for dehibilitated geriatric patients. Anabolic steriods antagonize certain undesirable effects of corticosteroids. Combined therapy of these with antirheumatic agents is sometimes desired. The anabolic possibility of Adroyd exceeds its androgenic potential to such an extent that, at recommended dosage, the masculinizing side-effects are generally no problem. Human tolerance studies so far have disclosed no prohibitive reactions to 30 to 60 mgs given for as long as four to six months.

Winstrol (stanozolol) is an anabolic energizer and a weak androgen (3). It was found by Beyler, Potts and Arnold (14) to have nearly thirty times the anabolic effect and about one-fourth the androgenic effect of methyltestosterone, a common reference androgen, when given orally.

For a review on anabolic therapy consult Berczeller and Kupperman (13) and Northington (42).

Spartase (potassium and magnesium aspartates). The use of Spartase is said to have shown a positive effect on athletics both in the reduction of existing fatigue and against the induction of fatigue. It is suggested for use in treating the tired patient who presents no evidence of organic dysfunction. Hicks (24) conducted an experimental study on 145 office patients, giving about half of them Spartase and the other approximate half placebos. Eighty-five per cent who received Spartase were positively affected, whereas only 9 per cent were helped who received the placebos. Shaw, Chesney, Tullis and Agersborg (53) reported effects on the use of Spartase in both physiologic and subjective tests on a series of 163 subjects. The two forms of tests corresponded well in both positive and negative effects. The prime effect was the relief of fatigue.

In an experiment on the swimming time of rats, Rosen, Blumenthal and Agersborg (49) found the animals with greater endurance were not improved by potassium and magnesium salts of aspartic acid, whereas the swmiming times of animals with the lesser endurance were prolonged.

In a study of ninety-two normal adults who complained of chronic fatigue, unabated by rest, Taylor (57) obtained a positive response in 80 per cent of the subjects. The study was a double-blind test in which thirty-six subjects received first the aspartates, and later the placebo, and seven received the placebo first and the aspartates last. In the subjects receiving placebos only, there were questionable to positive effects in 9 per cent. The 20 per cent failing to manifest benefit from the medication, were later examined and found to be suffering from anxiety and depression.

Among others reporting on the use of aspartates are Friedlander (19), Walkenstein, Bautillier, Wiser, and Alburn (59), Nussbaum (43), Kruse (30), and Crescente (15).

Improvement of Metabolism in General. One of the procedures often employed in dealing with fatigue and associated symptoms is the implementation of food intake with substance that are involved in general metabolism (see Table III). This often involves the administration of vitamins and minerals. The procedure is on the supposition that the diet is lacking in these necessary substances or that for some reason the individuals in question do not utilize these to the usual degree when present in the usual amounts. For example, it is quite common nowadays for certain patients to be given iron, calcium, and certain vitamins such as B_{12} by intramuscular injections. Some patients who exhibit deficiency symptoms even with what is ordinarily considered an adequate diet respond well to vitamin and mineral administration in this way. While these results are known to occur, the literature continues to assert that everyone on a varied diet is getting all the vitamins and minerals that are needed.

Iron therapy is one form of help for certain patients with fatigue, particularly those found to have anemia. This category may include a sizable number of geriatric patients.

One of the newer iron salts is a form of ferrous sulfate

(Feosal) given by capsules and sustained release capsules. Sterling (56) found this substance to have consistently milder and less frequent side effects than previously used forms of iron. It produced satisfactory rises in hemoglobin in all patients. Pegel (44) reported the same thing.

Pre-game Feeding of Athletes. The manufacturer of Sustagen has not made any advertising claims at this date regarding effect of subsequent fatigue, although it is conceivable that it may have beneficial effects in that direction.

Rose and Fuenning (47) have x-rayed athletes at various stages following eating and subsequent football playing. Pre-game tension in many cases was found to delay the emptying of the stomach and to reduce intestinal motility. This finding has a bearing upon the feeding of liquid diets before athletic contests, to aid in more prompt digestion and therefore promote the well-being of the subject. This ought to have considerable effect on performance and the onset of fatigue. The authors recommend two liquid protein hydrolysates, as Sustagen and Meritene.

Rose, Schneider and Sullivan (48) used Sustagen in a study on the effect of liquid pre-game meals for athletes. They found it eliminated pre-game nausea, and pre-game cramps, and improved strength and endurance.

Summary and Conclusion

It will have been noted that the drugs employed in combating fatigue or conditions which seem to underlie it have been classed into several categories: (1) those that relieve body discomfort, aspirin being the chief example on account of its analgesic, anti-rheumatic, and anti-anaphylactic properties; (2) those that improve muscle activity, caffeine being one of the best known substances; (3) those supposed to elevate mood, among which are the various ampetamines; (4) those classed definitely as anabolic energizers, though in some respects like the mood elevators; (5) the improvers of general metabolism less medicinal and extreme than the substances in the last group.

The question of what the complaint of fatigue means and what underlies it has been involved in the various choices of medicinals found in this chapter. Of all of the substances listed, the most of them were for use with patients either with long lasting chronic fatigue or for those recovering from illness, or for those whose fatigue is an outgrowth of tension and depression. Few, if any were strictly for normal subjects except those substances meant to aid in athletic events. The substances therefore were, for the most part, not meant for daily or even frequent use by so-called normal people, or at least outside of medical supervision.

CHAPTER SEVEN

The Management of Fatigue

OUR ATTENTION IN THIS CHAPTER WILL CENTER MAINLY OF FIVE CLASSES OF PERSONS AND WHAT to do for them. They are: (1) the normal or well individuals in the ordinary affairs of life; (2) those called upon to put forth extra exertion as in athletic contests; (3) those who present fatigue as a salient symptom in convalescence from illness; (4) patients who are frail and need some assistance; and (5) chronic fatigue patients who seem to be the victims of their own disorganized personalities.

The Normal Individual. Fatigue is something encountered by healthy people from time to time in everyday life. Part of it seems easily accounted for, because the victim can look back and remember that he performed some exertional task. So long as he can do this, the fatigue does not puzzle him and he goes his way and recovers. All to often, however, he cannot account for his fatigue. No heavy work was performed, and no other cause can be used to explain why he feels as he does.

In recent years, various standard verbalizations have come into use to supplement the idea that true fatigue is an energistic affair. For example, it is said that fatigue is emotional, i.e., it is caused by emotion. While this statement is used to explain fatigue, or to allay puzzlement, neither the speaker nor the listener has any conceptualization of emotion that would reasonably serve the purpose. Emotion is simply a feeling and emotional behavior is simply irratic behavior in which feeling is involved. The actual connection between this and fatigue is left unsolved. This being so, the would-be explainer is no further ahead than if he had kept quiet, except that he may *feel* that he has accomplished something.

At this point in our discussion it might be pertinent to say something about emotion. Again we find ourselves confronted with a word of many meanings. Again we can utilize its original meaning of the original class of phenomena that caused the word, emotion, to be used. When we do this, we indeed, find that emotions were feelings. For our purposes we must go beyond this and place these feelings into the activity structure of the human being. To account for these feelings, we must realize that the activities (responses) of the organism are always evaluative. They are selective. The orientation of the organism always determines which one of the possible alternative reactions it will make. This is true of complex sub-human organisms as well as the human.

The evaluation we refer to pertains to two things. It pertains to the organism's environment. Does the particular organism perceive the situation of the moment as threatening, as neutral, or as inviting and favorable. Naturally organisms, human or otherwise, do not verbalize as we have done here. Even the human evaluation is incipient, but no less real. The second thing evaluated by the organism, is its own reaction to the situation, in terms of the reaction called for. Neither is this evaluation the articulate kind that is expressed in words, but it is none the less real. This evaluative characteristic of behavior can be inferred by the expert observer from the way the organism behaves.

Where does emotion come in? It is to be explained as follows: When a human subject, for example, cannot react in the manner called for by the incipient and implicit evaluation involved, *substitute* activity takes the place of the *overt* and "adequate" reaction called for. These substitute reactions we have reference to are largely internal, involving disruptive effects in processes of the body and giving rise to feeling as one of the consequences.

Whatever is to be called emotional then is the expression of conflict between what the organism takes as *ought to be* and the situation *as is*.

Some people are quite permissive (relatively unselective) in the way they regard situations, and likewise they may be uncritical (relatively unselective) in what they expect of themselves. Other people range from this to being quite selective and then quite disturbed when things do not go their way, or when they cannot act in certain ways.

To the extent, then that being selective, and finding reality colliding with the value scale possessed, causes disorganization of internal body processes, this is likely to lead to various manifestations including emotion and fatigue.

Putting the matter as we have here is a long way from stopping with a pat statement that fatigue is sometimes emotional. What we have said describes the matter in such a way as to relate emotion to the disorganization we have described earlier as a basis for fatigue. It will be remembered that fatigue itself, with all the unpleasant awareness that it involves, was defined as an organically expressed evaluation of the individual's inability to cope with the demands of a task situation.

From the foregoing then, the normal person can be advised as to what fatigue is, what is consists in, and therefore what things to avoid that are not actually energistic affairs at all. Once the normal individual is able to grasp the explanation we have offered, he should not be puzzled about what makes him tired. He will simply know that whatever disorganizes him will likely cause him to end up tired, just as encountering the demands that make for muscle discomfort, or for depletion of energistic resources.

Athletic Performances. The following is a brief review of conclusions drawn with regard to a number of substances which have been used and/or advocated for improving athletic performance and forestalling fatigue.

As was stated earlier, the question of fatigue and the various factors influencing performance is one which interests men in athletics. The question of whether any substance fed to athletes will improve their performance and forestall fatigue has been of interest. Actually a certain amount of research has been done on the subject. It is not necessary here to discuss the various individual studies, however. It appears that negative results have attended most of the attempts to find such substances, or in cases in which decidedly positive results have been obtained they have been ruled out for use on medical and ethical grounds.

Alcohol. Alcohol has long been connected in various ways with the affairs of man. It has been so widely used in beverages that most everybody has an opinion about its uses and results. The question of whether it aids or hinders performance has not been overlooked. Various investigators have made tests of the effect of alcohol on energistic output. Diverse results have been obtained in experimental situations in keeping with amounts of alcohol taken, temporal relation between ingestion and work, habituation to alcohol, etc.

The ingestion of alcohol, like the taking of any other drug, produces a sequence of results. This temporal pattern is in keeping with the amounts taken, time of day, habituation etc. Accordingly positive effects in increasing work output can be shown under some conditions and for certain periods after ingestion. Sooner or later work output drops below par, so opinions differ as to whether alcohol may be utilized as a practical energy source for muscular work.

One thing is quite certain, most people do receive a pleasant effect from vasodilation and this is sometimes interpreted by the user as having "warmed up chilled muscles." The final conclusion to be pointed out here is that the regulation of amount of alcohol, the timing of its effects in relation to the work to be done is generally so tricky as to be of little use. One moment everything may seem to be advantageous and a little later benefits disappear. This swiftly changing sequence too often adds up to a definite net loss rather than a gain. What is needed is some substance whose beneficial effects, though not necessarily great at any instant will be maintained over a relatively long period and thus allow for some usable connection between the effect produced in the user and the work period that is involved.

In some countries, the custom of using weak wines and beer

is quite ingrained and we in this country may not rightly interpret the effects of alcohol on athletes from these countries.

Caffeine. Caffeine was mentioned in an earlier chapter.

Gelatine. Gelatine is high in aminoacetic acid, or glycine. This substance is closely related to creatine, a material needed for muscle contraction. On this account both gelatine and glycine have been tried for the improvement of muscle activity.

At first it was reported that glycine was beneficial to those with various muscular difficulties. It was said to decrease fatigability, i.e., increase work output. This result was reported for normals as well as for those below par. But later, better controlled investigations disclosed that some of the beneficial effects were results of training and not the gelatine.

In conclusion, it may be said that neither gelatine nor glycine have demonstrated their efficacy in proving muscle activity, either in strength or endurance. Hence we could say that these substances could be expected to have no detectable effect on fatigue.

Hormones. Various hormones, undoubtedly effect vital processes, such as increasing metabolism, raising blood pressure, insuring greater contractability of muscles. The lack of some of them, such as certain adrenal cortical substances, results in extreme muscular weakness. Some hormone substances have been tested, however, and have not shown that they increase work capacity. This was the case for Sympatol (oxyphenylethanol-methylamine).

At present generalized statements cannot be made for or against hormones, for the matter is too complex. It is probable, however, that the function of hormones is so subtle as not to be well utilized by the simple procedure of administering the hormones in standard doses in connection with athletic contests.

Fruit Juices. Fruit juices have had their advocates among those interested in improving muscular capacity, but experimental evidence indicates that, whatever good they are, they are not directly connected with processes providing improvement in muscular activity.

Sugar. Since it is known that sugar is fuel for muscular contraction, some advocates have given huge amounts of sugar to athletes, with the main result of causing gastric disturbances. The main physiological support for giving sugar has had to do with its use in prolonged exertion. Sugar given prior to required bursts of exertion is of no proven use.

Sodium Chloride. It has been thought that giving of sodium chloride would compensate for profuse sweating during severe exercise, and the known loss of sodium chloride incurred. Dill and associates (18) have shown the benefit of using sodium chloride in the form of tablets etc., to athletes where sweating is profuse. It must not be thought however, that sodium chloride adds anything to the energy output of muscle. It is usable only as a precautionary device against salt depletion in excessive sweating.

Lecithin. Lecithin is another substance that has had attention among those interested in improving metabolism during hard work. Lecithin is one of the phosphatids and contributes importantly to the oxidation of natural fats. Likewise it is a source of phosphorous involved in chemical changes in muscular contraction. Contrasting results have been achieved in its use in experimentation. It may be said with reference to lecithin, as in the case of many other substances, extra supply is redundant and does not lead to added utilization and the benefits expected.

Oxygen. The ubiquitous substance, oxygen, has naturally come in for examination with reference to improvement in muscular performance. Oxygen is one of the prime limiting factors in determining energistic activity. The organism can take up oxygen at only certain rates. It has seemed plausible that if pure oxygen is supplied, capacity for exertion and recovery from it would be enhanced. It has been found however, that breathing pure oxygen just before and just after a spurt of exertion is unnecessary. Forced breathing of air may be beneficial and will do just as well, some authorities believe.

Alkalies. Since during muscular activity, acids build up in the blood, it has been thought that increasing the supply of buffer alkalies in athletes would be helpful. Some evidence in this direction has been found, but there is also conflicting evidence. The net seems to be in favor of the idea that a judicious feeding of alkali such as sodium citrate, potassium citrate and sodium bicarbonate may do something toward improving muscular performance. There is, as yet, no knowledge as to what would be useful under competition conditions.

Cocaine. Cocaine has also been studied for its possible activating effect on muscular performance. The very earliest investigation on it in ergographic performance found it effective in increasing endurance. Others have found it speeded recovery from exertion. But since the substance is so dangerous as a narcotic and a habit-forming drug it is out of the question for use in this connection.

Coramine. Coramine, a stimulant of the central nervous system has been tested for its effects on certain athletic performance, in which case it seems beneficial at times, and not, at other times. No clear evidence has been presented in its favor. It stands as one of the drugs which if it did prove effective would likely be ruled out as unadvisable in competition athletes.

Digitalis. Digitalis, owing to the fact that it effects the heart, has been suggested as helpful in exertional performance such as athletics. The same thing can be said about its inadvisability in competitive athletics as for Coramine.

Metrazol. Metrazol (pentamethylenetetrazol) a drug affecting the vasomotor and respiratory cortex has been used on subjects in a variety of exertional activities such as mountain climbing, bicycling, hiking, etc. It has seemingly improved endurance in some of these situations. These were not controlled experiments however. Again, it must be cautioned that the use of such drugs in competitive sports would hardly be countenanced, even if shown to be effective on performance.

It can be concluded that the management of fatigue and work output in athletics should not depend to any great extent on drugs and special substances that are advocated to aid in metabolic processes. Athletes either don't need such substances in the first place, or else if perchance they may be effective, feeding is ruled out on much the same grounds as feeding cocaine to race horses. It is dangerous, unfair, and unpredictable.

Amphetamine. More recently several groups naturally interested in athletics and human performance under conditions demanding extremes of exertion have become interested in the question of whether the amphetamines, commonly dubbed as "pep pills" do actually improve athletes performance. A special committee of the American Medical Association aided by certain other groups looked into the matter. One of the initial questions was whether the amphetamines had been used by athletes in this country in their contests. They found that athletic organizations had not used the drugs and that their leaders had strongly condemned their use.

In addition there was no well-established evidence in the literature that the amphetamines did improve athletic performance. H. K. Beecher (54), a member of the *ad hoc* Committee of the American Medical Association on Amphetamines and Athletes, volunteered to make an experimental study on the subject. About this time it was discovered that Dr. P. V. Karpovich had already projected a study of the same kind. These studied were carried out and we now have information on the question of what to expect of amphetamines in athletic situations.

In what follows, we shall briefly review the results.

Karpovich (29) studied the following activities: (1) running to exhaustion on a treadmill at 7.2 mph at a 5 degree tilt with a ten minute rest between runs; (2) swimming 100 yards at maximum speeds twice in succession, with a ten minute rest interval between; (3) swimming 220 and 440 yards once per test day; (4) running 220 yards outdoors for time trials; and (5) running various distances (100 yards to 2 miles) under competition. All of the laboratory type experiments consisted of six trials on six different occasions, three with amphetamine and three with placebos.

All subjects were males in college. Most swimmers and all the track men were on the varsity teams. Twenty-five men were tested on the treadmills, eighteen were used in swimming, and eleven were used in track.

In the first part of the study (1958) all but four were given 10 mg of amphetamine sulphate an hour before testing. Neither

Karpovich nor his assistants knew at the time which subjects received the drug and which received the placebo.

In 1959, all subjects were given 20 mg of amphetamine or the placebo thirty minutes before testing. In all cases the placebo was calcium lactate.

Subjective reports were asked of the subjects. These had to do with reporting any unusual sensations and whether they slept well or not. This was not actually a direct fatigue report. At least nothing could be gained from Karpovich's article dealing with fatigue by name. It was found that with the 10 mg capsules and the placebos, both were praised or discounted equally often. When 20 mg of the drug or placebos were given, the subjects guessed correctly 75 per cent of the time. Some subjects reported difficulty in sleeping. The four subjects in a special treadmill group generally reported correctly when given the amphetamine. One subject from India who had never used any drugs in his life was able to report correctly in every case. His running was the same with and without the drug.

The performance results were as follows: Only four subjects out of the fifty-four showed either beneficial or harmful results from use of the amphetamine either in the 10 or 20 mg doses. Three of the four markedly improved in their 220 swim, and one improved in the 440 swim. One treadmill subject ran longer in the placebo condition than in the drug condition. All of the men showing either beneficial or harmful effects of amphetamine had been given the 20 mg doses.

Smith and Beecher (54) conducted the following investigation. In plannnig the investigation they were aware that a number of variables might be involved in determining the effect of amphetamine on athletic performance. Among the factors thought likely were: dosage, time after dosage before testing performance; fatigue state of subject, type of athletic event (short and intense versus less intense and prolonged), dependence upon form of performance as well as upon strength, whether competition was with time or with another athlete, expectations concerning drug; mood of subject, whether in top form or not, and whether highly motivated or not. This list looks like a pretty good array of considerations.

The performances studied were swimming, running and weight throwing. Six experiments were performed. Each differed in pattern of variables, and each experiment was separately reported upon. The details of the experimental conditions etc., are too numerous to describe here.

All subjects in all six conditions received 14 mg of amphetamine sulphate per 70 kg of body weight, and placebos. The experiments were conducted on a double-blind basis. Other medicaments were used as experimental variables in some cases.

The results showed that all three classes of athletes (swimmers, runners, and weight-throwers) performed better under amphetamine than with placebos. From 67 to 93 per cent of the swimmers, depending upon conditions tested, performed better; 73 per cent of the runners, and 85 per cent of the weight-throwers performed better. The percentage improvement was not great in absolute amount but in terms of competitive significance it was sizable, and it was statistically significant.

Since the use of any drug to enhance athletic performance has been the basis for disqualification by the Amateur Athletic Union. the International Amateur Athletic Federation and The United States Olympic Association, the Committee of the American Medical Association on Amphetamine and Athletics recommended that the use of amphetamines be condemned for this purpose.

Now we seem to have the answer. Amphetamines do activate trained athletes, but the use of such drugs is definitely tabooed for this purpose. The same taboo, of course, would not be extended to substances that are not drugs, but are simply nutritional. However, there are other substances, those that could be classified as neither items of nutrition nor those artificially activating the individual in the amphetamine manner. Their place in athletics, if effective, has not yet been morally determined.

Fatigue in Prolonged Convalescents. A number of patients who complain of fatigue are those who feel quite inadequate and forget that not too long ago they were the victims of some infectious or otherwise debilitating disease. This fact must be taken into account in managing fatigue in such individuals. The assumption underlying the management is that they are not always going to be in the below-par condition they manifest now. Their treatment is no transient affair but neither is it the perpetual affair that underlies some conditions such as hypothyroidism, for example. The question arises therefore whether there are medications useful in alleviating the fatigue such patients complain of.

The preceding chapter contained a sampling of some of the opinions of physicians regarding the various pharmaceuticals on the market intended for fatigue alleviation. It will have been evident that both pro and con reports are to be found for a number of such substances. Actually many of the substances in this category are relatively new. That is, they are among the many medicinals whose usage will improve with a much larger period of experience with them. Further improvement in their usage will come also from a clearer diagnosis and categorization of patients who come to the physician with the primary complaint of fatigue.

It is said that a great fraction of the patients complaining of fatigue are psychoneurotic. Other writers, of course, lean on the somatic origin represented in convalescence from debilitating disease. Some point out that the results of chemotherapy alone have not been too encouraging (61). Some remind us of the fact that one significant cause of fatigue in depressed patients is a derangement of carbohydrate metabolism expressed in a more or less chronic state of hypoglycemia. Since the brain is dependent upon sugar for its normal functioning a short supply brings about central nervous malfunction as well as muscular difficulty. The symptoms of hypoglycemia depend more upon the speed with which blood sugar level drops than with actual concentrations (within certain range). On this account a slow lowering of blood sugar level often is not accompanied by the expected symptoms. Under some conditions, certain cases of hypoglycemia will be missed in checking for it. Some writers describe what is called psychogenic hypoglycemia. A number of cases of chronic hypoglycemia in connection with mental depression have been reported. The attacks of depression as they recurred showed hypoglycemia symptoms. Strangely enough these episodes were mostly postprandial, at a time when blood sugar level should have been at maximum. Treatment directed toward the psychic (personalistic) symptoms abolished the hypoglycemia symptoms. Among patients treated with orange juice and sugar to bolster blood sugar level, some are helped, and some show an increase in hypoglycemia symptoms. Kamman (28) suggests a way of inhibiting pancreatic secretions of insulin by atropine sulphate, three times a day, one-half hour before meals. He believes this is helpful in certain types of hypoglycemia.

His advice, however, for treating fatigue is to not rely on medicine alone, but to use "rational psychotherapy," physiotherapy, diet, occupational and recreational therapy. In fact he suggests carrying out an "intelligent management of the patient's life as a whole."

The assumption we are making is that some metabolic help is needed by the class of patients we are including here, but that in addition to whatever medication is involved, some recognition of the interrelatedness of the phenomena at the biochemical or organ-system level and the organization of the individual as a total must be made. Anytime that the two classes of phenomena, the personalistic and the biochemical, are separated as if independent, failure is likely.

Frail Patients. In the preceding section, patients convalescing from disease were discussed. Many included were those presenting symptoms of depression, and many forms of depression are akin to psychoneurosis. Perhaps not all depressed patients have a history of infection and disease as an origin for their depression and fatigue, but for our purpose those that have not had such a history can be classed with those that have had.

Now we are coming to the class of frail individuals who may not be depressed in particular but who still tire easily. What is to be done for them? This class includes individuals in the older age ranges, and others who through a sedentary life do not manifest much physical fitness. Three kinds of situations are particularly important in connection with these individuals.

Requirements calling for expenditure of extra exertion, prolonged tasks and situations that distract and disturb. Individuals in this general category may be classed in several ways: (1) those who go along quietly and routinely if left to themselves; (2) those who manufacture their own disorganization; (3) those with a material amount of muscular and joint or circulatory disability. Most of these people should not judge themselves by the standards applying to normal people, nor should others judge them by such criteria.

The effectiveness of such people is not commensurate with the hours spent at work, but rather with the control they have over themselves and their affairs so as to move at their own pace, and vary their activities in accord with the tension and fatigue they develop while at any given task, and with avoidance of distraction.

The Chronic Fatigue Patient. Such individuals have been mentioned already in a manner implying how they are to be regarded but there are some generalizations which are appropriate here.

Chronic fatigue, in the broad sense of the word, is any fatigue that lingers from day to day over a prolonged period. It may be possible to distinguish between two forms, the fatigue in which the patient still finds himself weak and unable to carry on as he expects, and the fatigue that haunts the person who has a disordered outlook on life and has a set of habits which reflects this. If one can be sure that he in confronting a patient in this category he can proceed in a different way than in dealing with a patient in the first category.

Most all people when they experience fatigue for extended periods expect that there is or should be some medication which if used would alleviate it and restore them to vigor and adequacy. Probably the main thing that the patient in question needs is to be convinced that his troubles lie in his personal disorganization; or to say the least, in some sort of unrealistic expectation regarding himself and not in some specific "medical" affliction. The demonstration that this is the case is no easy accomplishment. Here again, the lingering outmoded and inadequate mind-body dualism inherent in everyday thinking is a decided drawback. For according to that outlook, one's troubles are either in his *body* or in his *mind,* and the victim is absolutely certain that his troubles (fatigue) are not in his mind. To talk to him about attitudes and belief is to seem to be talking to him about something that is not quite real, and to be misunderstanding and belittling the significance of the matter. It hasn't been long since physicians themselves have meant to be minimizing the matter in telling the patient his troubles are "in his head." They well knew that they had no effective medication for the ailment, and may have been annoyed by the class of patient they were having to deal with.

The management of fatigue is to be achieved from the efforts of two persons, advisor and/or physicians, and the fatigue victim himself. There are some things that need to be done that the victim already knows ought to be done. With reference to these the victim needs confirmation and encouragement and some boosting in order that they actually get done. There are other things that only the person along side the victim can do. Very often it is not so much what needs to be done, as the doing of it that is problematic. In fact, any discussion of hygiene etc., is likely to sound quite preachy, but it is not apparent how this can be avoided.

There are five different types of things that may be involved in the management of fatigue: (1) some clarification as to what fatigue is and then what it is that is to be dealt with and achieved; (2) the treatment of disease, if present. This, of course, is determined and dealt with by first submitting to a physical examination. (3) The establishment of a reasonable physiological hygiene which, for example, may consist in the following: (a) an activity rest cycle suitable for the particular individual involved. Such a cycle is certainly not the same for all persons, but the determination of what is suitable for the person involved in a worthwhile procedure; (b) the temperate use of stimulants, and alcohol; (c) the elimination of any chronic self-medication that may have become habitual, though not wholly believed in by the person himself; (d) the use of warm and cold baths to produce relaxation and toning; (e) the regulation of eating times and the avoidance of foods that may not be well tolerated; (f) the possible use of formal physiotherapy; (g) the development of a program of exercise to develop a better cardio-circulatory system. The absence of habitual exercise results in a demonstrable sympathetic-adrenergic preponderance in the neurovegatative regulative of cardiac activity at rest. This is in contrast with the vagotonic or sympatho-inhibitory characteristics displayed by the physically fit. The patient himself will not know objectively when he is accomplishing this shift but the sophisticated observer or physician can determine by test if need be.

(4) Another factor is the discarding of habits of either hurry or of indolence and sluggishness. One habitual feature of people's behavior consists in reacting too violently to the minute-by-minute events that occur around them and in that way undergoing more disorganization and daily wear and tear than is necessary. (5) The development of an improved and more wholesome outlook on life in general. This is certainly a helpful factor in reducing fatigue.

References

1. Alexander, L.: Chemotherapy of depression—use of meprobamate combined with benactyzine (2-diethylaminoethyl benzilate) hydrochloride. *J.A.M.A.*, *166*:1019, 1958.
2. Alvarez, W. C.: What is the matter with the patient who is chronically tired; *J. Missouri M. A.*, *38*:365-368, 1941.
3. Arnold, A., Beyler, A. L., and Potts, G. O.: Andro-stranazole, a new orally active anabolic steriod. *Proc. Soc. Exp. Biol. Med.*, *102*:184, 1959.
4. Bartley, S. H.: Conflict, frustration and fatigue. *Psychosom. Med.*, *5*:160-162, 1943.
5. Bartley, S. H., and Chute, E.: A preliminary clarification of the concept of fatigue. *Psychol. Rev.*, *53*:169-174, 1945.
6. Bartley, S. H., and Chute, E.: *Fatigue and Impairment in Man.* New York, McGraw-Hill, 1947.
7. Bartley, S. H.: The basis of visual fatigue. *Amer. J. Optom. Monogr. No. 30*, 1947.
8. Bartley, S. H.: *Fatigue and Efficiency in Theoretical Foundations of Psychology.* H. Helson (ed.), New York, Van Nostrand, 1951.
9. Bartley, S. H.: Understanding visual fatigue. *Amer. J. Optom.*, *31*:29-40, 1954.
10. Bartley, S. H.: Fatigue, aspirations and conflicting demands. *Kitchen Reports.* (Feb.) 1955.
11. Bartley, S. H.: Fatigue and inadequacy. *Physiol. Revs.*, *37*:301-324, 1957.
12. Beerman, H. M.: The treatment of depression with meprobamate benactyzine HC1. *Western Med.*, *1*:10, 1960.
13. Berczeller, P. H., and Kapperman, H. S.: The anabolic steroids. *Clin. Pharmacol. Therap.*, *1*:464, 1960.
14. Beyler, A. L., Potts, G. O., and Arnold, A.: Anabolic properties of androstane—[3, 2-c]—pyrozoles. Presented at meeting of Endocrine Society. Atlantic City (June) 1959.

15. Cresente, F. J.: Treatment of fatigue in a surgical practice. *J. Abdom. Surg., 4*:73-76, 1962.

16. DaCosta, J. M.: On irritable heart: a clinical study of a form of functional cardiac disorder and its consequences. *Amer. J. Med. Sci., 61*:17-52, 1871.

17. Dill, D. B., Bock, A. V., Edwards, H. T., and Kennedy, P. H.: Industrial fatigue. *J. Indust. Hyg. Toxicol., 18*:417, 1936.

18. Edwards, H. T., Thorndike, A., and Dill, D. B.: The energy requirement in strenuous exercise. *N. England J. Med., 213*:532, 1935.

19. Friedlander, H. S.: Fatigue as a presenting symptom: management in general practice. *Curr. Therap. Res., 4*:443-449, 1962.

20. Gearren, J. B.: Trifluoperazine in emotionally disturbed office patients. *Dis. Nerv. Syst., 20*:66-68 (Feb.) 1959.

21. Gordon, P. E.: Deprol in the treatment of depression. *Dis. Nerv. Syst., 21*:215, 1960.

22. Gross, I. H., and Bartley, S. H.: Fatigue in house care. *J. Appl. Psychol., 35*:205-207, 1951.

23. Harms, H. E., and Soniat, T. L. L.: The meaning of fatigue. *Med. Clin. N. Amer., 36*:311-317, 1952.

24. Hicks, J. T.: Treatment of fatigue in general practice: double blind study. *Clin. Med., 71*:85-90, 1964.

25. Himwich, H. E.: *Stimulants in the Effect of Pharmacological Agents on the Nervous System.* F. J. Braceland (ed.), Baltimore, Williams & Wilkins, 1959, p. 356-385.

26. Hollingworth, H. L.: The influence of caffeine on mental and motor efficiency. *Arch. Psychol., 22*:1-66, 1912.

27. Immerman, S. L.: What constitutes neurocirculatory asthenia. *J. Aviat. Med., 12*:236-239, 1941.

28. Kamman, G. R.: Fatigue as a symptom in depressed patients. *J. Lancet.,* 238-240 (July) 1945.

29. Karpovich, P. V.: Effect of amphetamine sulfate on athlete's performance. *J. A. M. A., 170*:558-561, 1959.

30. Kruse, C. A.: Treatment of fatigue with aspartic acid salts. *North West Med., 60*:597-603, 1961.

31. Lemere, F., and Lasater, J. H.: Deanol (Deaner) in the treatment of neurasthemia and mild depression. *Amer. J. Psychiat., 114*:655, 1958.

32. Lemere, F.: Pharmacologic treatment of depression. *Northwestern Med., 57*:1149-1150, 1958.

33. Lewis, T.: The Soldier's Heart and the Effort Syndrome. New

York (Paul B. Hoeber, Inc.), Harper & Bros., 1920, p. 144.

34. Maerz, J. C., Lee, H. G., and Hunter, H. H.: Psychosomatic disorders treated with trifluoperazine. *Psychosom. Med., 111*:220-222, 1962.

35. May, A. R., Whitely, J. S., and Gradwell, B. G.: Trifluoperazine (Stelazine) in psychoneuroses: A clinical assessment. *J. Ment. Dis., 105*:1059-1063, 1959.

36. McClure, C. W.: Workshop Study on Depression, in Depression and Antidepressant Drugs. D. M. Rogers (ed.) Metropolitan State Hospital, Massachusetts Department of Mental Health, Waltham, 1960, p. 38-45.

37. Meller, R. L.: Treatment of mild depression with Deanol Paraacetamidobenzoate. *J. Lancet, 79*:25-26, 1959.

38. Moriarty, J. D., and Mebane, J. C.: Clinical experiences with deanol (Deaner): a different kind of Psychic energizer. *J. Neuropsychiat., 1*:1-2, 1959.

39. Moriarty, J. D., and Mebane, J. D.: Clinical uses of deanol (Deanor) a new type of psychotropic drug. *Amer. J. Psychiat., 115*:941-942, 1959.

40. Muncie, W.: Chronic fatigue. *Psychosom. Med., 3*:277-285, 1941.

41. Muscio, B.: Is a fatigue test possible? *Brit. J. Psychol., 12*:31-46, 1921-22.

42. Northington, J. M.: Present state of an anabolic therapy. *Clin. Med., 7*:1115, 1960.

43. Nussbaum, H. E.: Chronic fatigue. *J. Med. Soc. New Jersey, 60*:499-503, 1963.

44. Pegel, L. A.: Iron therapy for aged patients. *J. Amer. Geriat. Soc., 6*:621-622, 1958.

45. Rickels, K., and Ewing, J. H.: Deprol in depressive conditions. *Dis. Nerv. Syst., 20*:364, 1959.

46. Robey, W. H., and Boas, E. P.: Neurocirculatory asthenia. *J. A. M. A., 71*:525-529, 1918.

47. Rose, K. D., and Fuenning, S. I.: Pre-game emotional tension, gastrointestinal motility and the feeding of athletes. *Nebraska Med. J., 45*:575-579, 1960.

48. Rose, K. D., Schneider, P. J., and Sullivan, R. P. T.: A liquid pre-game meal for athletes. *J. A. M. A., 178*:30-33, 1961.

49. Rosen, H., Blumenthal, A., and Agersborg, H. P. K.: Effects of potassium and magnesium salts of asportic acid on metabolic exhaustion. *J. Pharmaceut. Sci., 51*:592-593, 1962.

50. Rowell, S. S., and Segall, M. L. J.: The treatment of psycho-

neurotic symptoms with trifluoperazine in general practice. *Practitioner, 184*:235-238, 1960.
51. Selye, H.: *Stress of Life.* New York, McGraw-Hill, 1956.
52. Settel, E. S.: Stimulant therapy with Deanol in depression, migraine and tension headaches. *J. Amer. Geriat. Soc.,* 7:877-879, 1959.
53. Shaw, D. L., Chesney, M. S., Tullis, I. F., and Agersborg, H. P. K.: Management of fatigue: A physiologic approach. *Amer. J. Med. Sci., 243*:98-108, 1964.
54. Smith, G. M., and Beecher, H. K.: Amphetamine sulfate and athletes performance. *J. A. M. A., 170*:542-557, 1959.
55. Snow, E. W., Machlow, L. O., Warnell, C. E., and Utt, T. P.: The tired patient. *Med. Times* (Nov.) 1959.
56. Sterling, M. P.: Summary of three years clinical experience with a new form of ferrous sulfate. *J. Amer. Med. Wom. Ass., 15*:971-973, 1960.
57. Taylor, B. B.: The fatigued worker. *Western Med., 2*:535-538, 1961.
58. Tracy, F. E.: The cyclic psychosomatic fatigue syndrome. *Conn. Med., 24*:357-359, 1960.
59. Walkenstein, S. S., Bautillier, E., Wiser, R., and Alburn, H. E.: Screening antifatigue agents by radio respirometry. *J. Pharmaceut. Sci., 51*:598-599, 1962.
60. Whiting, H. F., and English, H. B.: Fatigue tests and incentives. *J. Exp. Psychol., 8*:33-48, 1925.
61. Wilbur, D. L.: Clinical management of the patient with fatigue and nervousness. *J. A. M. A., 141*:1199-1204, 1949.
62. Wittkower, E., Roger, T. F., and Wilson, A. T. M.: Effort syndrome. *J. Lancet, 1*:531-535, 1941.
63. Young, Z. O.: Deaner, a new stimulant for office practice. *Clin. Med.,* 6 (October) 1959.

Tables

TABLE I

AMPHETAMINES

Trade Name	Chemical Name
Adjudets	racemic amphetamine phosphate
Ambar	methamphetamine plus phenobarbital
Amphedase	d-amphetamine sulfate
	niacinamide
	thiamine hydrochloride
	aspergillus oryzae enzymes
Amphedroxyn	multifactor methamphetamine hydrochloride
Amphedroxyn (hydrochloride)	methamphetamine hydrochloride
Benzedrine	amphetamine sulfate
Biphetamine	resin complexes of d and dl amphetamine
Biphetamine-T	resin complexes of d and dl amphetamine plus methaqualone
Dexamyl	
Dexedrine	d-amphetamine sulfate
Drinalfa	methamphetamine hydrochloride
Methedrine	amphetamine hydrochloride
Obocell	d-amphetamine phosphate (dibasic)
Obocell TF=	d-amphetamine phosphate (dibasic) plus methapyrilene plus methylcellulose
Raphetamine	racemic amphetamine phosphate
Synatan	d-amphetamine tannate
Syndrox	methamphetamine hydrochloride

TABLE II

SUBSTANCES (EXCLUDING AMPHETAMINES) ACTING ON THE CENTRAL NERVOUS SYSTEM

Trade Name	Chemical Name	Function
Elavil	amitriptyline hydrochloride plus dextrose, Methylparaben propylparaben in aquous solution for injection	both anti-depressant and tranquilizer
Deaner	deanol (para-acetamidobenzoic acid salt of 2-dimethylaminoethanol)	psychic energizer
Deprol	Benactyzine (2-diethylaminoethyl benzilate hydrochloride) meprobamate	both anti-depressant and tranquilizer
? (not yet on market)	nortriptyline	non-sympathomimetic anti-depressant
Ritalin	(methylphenidate hydrochloride)	anti-depressant
Stelazine	trifluoperazine	central nervous depressant

TABLE III

IRON, MINERALS, VITAMINS, ETC.

Trade Name	*Composition and/or Use*
Feosol capsules	Oral sustained-release iron preparation (ferrous sulfate)
Troph-Iron	B_{12}, B_1, vitamins, elemental iron
Eskay's Neurophosphates	Strychnine, sodium glycerolphosphate, calcium glycerolphosphate, phosphoric acid
Vi-Sorbin	B_{12}, B_6, Ferric pyrophosphate, folic acid
Zentinic	Multifactor hematinic with vitamins
Zentron	Iron, vitamin B complex, vitamin C
Eskay's Theranates	Alcohol, B^1 vitamin, strychnine, sodium glycerolphosphate, calcium glycerolphosphate, phosphoric acid
Pre-Mens tablets	A diuretic, a stimulant (caffeine alkaloid) vitamin B complex
Eldec	Vitamins, minerals, digestive enzymes; basic gonadal hormones
Liquid Potassium Triplex	For replacement therapy in fatigue due to loss of electrolyte balance

MISCELLANEOUS

Adroyd	Oxymetholone, a strong anabolic, a weak androgenic
Spartase	Potassium and magnesium aspartates, helpful in intermediate metabolism
Sustagen	Liquid pre-game meal for athletes
Winstrol	Stanozolol, a strong anabolic, a weak androgenic

Index